IAP

PEDIATR

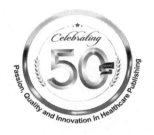

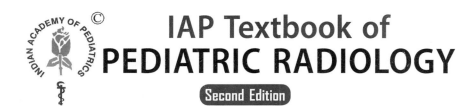

IAP Textbook of
PEDIATRIC RADIOLOGY

Second Edition

Editors-in-Chief

TM Ananda Kesavan
MD (Pediatrics) DNB MNAMS FIAP FIAMS FRCP (Edinburgh) PGDDN
(Postgraduate Diploma in Developmental Neurology)
Additional Professor
Department of Pediatrics
Government Medical College
Thrissur, Kerala, India

S Venkateswaran
MD (Pediatrics) DCH DMRD
Former Professor of Pediatrics
Madurai Medical College
Former Chief-in-Charge of Division of Neonatology
Institute of Child Health and Research Center
Madurai Medical College and
Government Rajaji Hospital
Madurai, Tamil Nadu, India

Editors

Mona D Shastri
MD (Radiodiagnosis)
Professor and Head
Department of Radiodiagnosis
SMIMER
Surat, Gujarat, India

G Vijayalakshmi DMRD DNB PhD
Professor and HOD
Department of Pediatric
Radiology and Imaging
Institute of Child Health &
Hospital for Children
Chennai, Tamil Nadu, India

Anoop Verma
MD FIAP FCGP FIAMS FPAI
Director
Swapnil Institute of Child Health
Raipur, Chhattisgarh, India

M Zulfikar Ahamed
MBBS DCH MD (Pediatrics)
DM (Cardiology)
Senior Consultant Pediatric
Cardiologist
KIMS Hospital
Thiruvananthapuram
Professor of Cardiology
Pushpagiri Medical College, Thiruvalla
Clinical Professor of
Pediatric and Adolescent Cardiology
Child Development Center
Thiruvananthapuram, Kerala, India

Anand S Vasudev
DNB DPed MNAMS FIAP FIMSA
Senior Consultant, Pediatric Nephrology
Department of Pediatrics
Indraprasth Apollo Hospital,
Max Hospital
New Delhi, India

TK Nandakumaran MBBS MS MCh
Professor
Department of Pediatric Surgery
Government Medical College
Kannur, Kerala, India

Manish Kumar MD (Pediatrics)
ISPN Fellow Pediatric Nephrology
Associate Professor
Department of Pediatrics
Chacha Nehru Bal Chikitsalaya
Delhi, India

Kavita Menghani MBBS DCH
Consultant Pediatrician
Dr Kavita Menghani Clinic
Raipur, Chhattisgarh, India

Pulak Parag MS (General Surgery)
MCh (Pediatric Surgery)
(Freelance) Senior Consultant
Pediatric Surgery
Raipur, Chhattisgarh, India

Executive Editors

TU Sukumaran
MD MNAMS FIAP MPhil PhD
Head, Department of Pediatrics
Pushpagiri Institute of Medical Sciences
Thiruvalla, Kerala, India

Digant D Shastri
MD (Pediatrics) FIAP PGDHHM
President, Indian Academy of Pediatrics
Member, Standing Committee
International Pediatric Association 2019-21
Managing Editor
Asia Pacific Journal of Pediatrics and Child Health
Mumbai, Maharashtra, India

Foreword
Digant D Shastri

JAYPEE BROTHERS MEDICAL PUBLISHERS
The Health Sciences Publisher
New Delhi | London

Jaypee Brothers Medical Publishers (P) Ltd

Headquarters
Jaypee Brothers Medical Publishers (P) Ltd
4838/24, Ansari Road, Daryaganj
New Delhi 110 002, India
Phone: +91-11-43574357
Fax: +91-11-43574314
Email: jaypee@jaypeebrothers.com

Overseas Office
J.P. Medical Ltd
83, Victoria Street, London
SW1H 0HW (UK)
Phone: +44 20 3170 8910
Fax: +44 (0)20 3008 6180
E-mail: info@jpmedpub.com

Website: www.jaypeebrothers.com
Website: www.jaypeedigital.com

IAP Textbook of Pediatric Radiology

First Edition: 2013

Second Edition: **2020**

ISBN: 978-93-89188-97-4

Printed at Sanat Printers

Dedicated to

*All those stalwarts of Indian Academy of Pediatrics,
who strived hard and relentlessly to build the organization to international standard.*

Contributors

Anand S Vasudev DNB DPed MNAMS FIAP FIMSA
Senior Consultant, Pediatric Nephrology
Department of Pediatrics
Indraprasth Apollo Hospital, Max Hospital
New Delhi, India

Anoop Verma MD FIAP FCGP FIAMS FPAI
Director
Swapnil Institute of Child Health
Raipur, Chhattisgarh, India

G Vijayalakshmi DMRD DNB PhD
Professor and HOD
Department of Pediatric Radiology and
Imaging
Institute of Child Health &
Hospital for Children
Chennai, Tamil Nadu, India

Kavita Menghani MBBS DCH
Consultant Pediatrician
Dr Kavita Menghani Clinic
Raipur, Chhattisgarh, India

M Zulfikar Ahamed
MBBS DCH MD (Pediatrics) DM (Cardiology)
Senior Consultant Pediatric Cardiologist
KIMS Hospital, Thiruvananthapuram
Professor of Cardiology
Pushpagiri Medical College, Thiruvalla
Clinical Professor of
Pediatric and Adolescent Cardiology
Child Development Center
Thiruvananthapuram, Kerala, India

Manish Kumar MD (Pediatrics)
ISPN Fellow Pediatric Nephrology
Associate Professor
Department of Pediatrics
Chacha Nehru Bal Chikitsalaya
Delhi, India

Mona D Shastri MD (Radiodiagnosis)
Professor and Head
Department of Radiodiagnosis
SMIMER
Surat, Gujarat, India

Pulak Parag
MS (General Surgery) MCh (Pediatric Surgery)
(Freelance) Senior Consultant
Pediatric Surgery
Raipur, Chhattisgarh, India

S Venkateswaran MD (Pediatrics) DCH DMRD
Former Professor of Pediatrics
Madurai Medical College
Former Chief-in-Charge of
Division of Neonatology
Institute of Child Health and
Research Center
Madurai Medical College and
Government Rajaji Hospital
Madurai, Tamil Nadu, India

TK Nandakumaran MBBS MS MCh
Professor
Department of Pediatric Surgery
Government Medical College
Kannur, Kerala, India

TM Ananda Kesavan MD (Pediatrics) DNB
MNAMS FIAP FIAMS FRCP (Edinburgh) PGDDN
(Postgraduate Diploma in Developmental Neurology)
Additional Professor
Department of Pediatrics
Government Medical College
Thrissur, Kerala, India

TU Sukumaran MD MNAMS FIAP MPhil PhD
Head, Department of Pediatrics
Pushpagiri Institute of Medical Sciences
Thiruvalla, Kerala, India

Foreword

Indeed it is proud privilege for me to write the foreword for the 2nd Edition of *IAP Textbook of Pediatric Radiology*.

Recent growth in the field of diagnostic radiology has dramatically increased the complexity of this field. Diagnostic imaging has become widely available and plays an increasing role in diagnosis and therapy.

With availability of many modalities and availability of radiology facilities at district and taluka places at time it is found that it leads to the ordering of incorrect imaging studies, duplication of orders, unnecessary requests for follow-up imaging, too many exam orders, and other problems. The risk of radiation hazard is also to be kept in mind while submitting children for any radiological investigations.

Child health and well-being are the core areas of mission statement of Indian Academy of Pediatrics and for that IAP is involved in knowledge upgradation of pediatricians through organizing CMEs, conferences, workshops and publishing books. Earlier IAP Textbook of Pediatric Radiology was published in 2013 and was found to be very successful and popular amongst pediatricians. With the recent growth in the field of diagnostic radiology, it was necessary to publish the second edition of IAP Textbook of Pediatric Radiology.

As president of IAP I am happy that editorial team led by Dr TM Ananda Kesavan and Dr S Venkateswaran worked hard to bring this second edition. The book is written, with general pediatricians in mind, as an alternative to the traditionally large (and hard to learn) reference textbooks. This book does not detail the literature of all disease processes. Instead, it is focused on the most common clinical scenarios encountered in daily practice. It also includes practical imaging techniques and protocols used to address common problems, and can give readers easily accessible tools to aid in reaching a specific diagnosis.

I congratulate the editorial team and contributors and thank them for their contribution. I am sure it will be proved as one of the most popular publications of IAP.

Digant D Shastri MD (Pediatrics) FIAP PGDHHM
President, Indian Academy of Pediatrics
Member, Standing Committee
International Pediatric Association 2019-21
Managing Editor
Asia Pacific Journal of Pediatrics and Child Health
Mumbai, Maharashtra, India

Preface to the Second Edition

"Retain the past and Refresh with new" is the concept we have adopted in this edition. Since the first edition is a Master edition with the excellent proposition of chapters and topics, the essential style and format have been retained and we have added few interesting topics and case scenarios. As a face lifting to previous edition, Dr Mona D Shastri has presented an excellent start up writing about the discovery and evolution of X-rays. Also she has given an outline of radiation hazards, types of X-rays and most important radiographic positions in pediatrics which is easy to understand by any pediatrician. Since the X-ray chest is the most commonly utilized investigation, the advent of Digital chest X-ray and respiratory clinical case scenarios added by Dr S Venkateswaran is an important practical addition in this text. The cardiovascular system by Dr M Zulfikar Ahamed is face lifted by addition of interesting X-rays and cases. The add up cases in Bone and Metabolic diseases by Dr G Vijayalakshmi elevates the chapter to completion. The additional insertion of case scenarios by Dr TM Ananda Kesavan adds color to this edition.

Although many of us are comfortable with new imaging modalities and contemporary techniques, it is not possible with all the patients and with all the pediatricians. The approach in this book provides an effective and cost containing evaluation in a medical environment beset with financial constraints and unfamiliar imaging modalities. For this reason, the text is additionally and especially suited to pediatricians practicing primary care pediatrics and emergency room pediatrics.

We have tried to limit all changes to those that are truly significant in a practical sense, rather than change for the sake of change. It is our hope and belief that a pediatrician with the content of this book will be able to approach sick children professionally with skill and confidence. We hope that this book meets our goals, and we remain grateful for any comments and criticisms that our readers may wish to offer.

TM Ananda Kesavan
S Venkateswaran

Preface to the First Edition

The aim of this Textbook of Pediatric Radiology is to provide valid and vibrant information to practicing pediatricians at all levels especially who are dealing with level one care.

It is an undeniable fact that pediatric radiology differs from adult radiology and many a time even many of the general radiologists and even few of the so called pediatric radiologist may find it difficult to interpret and may feel uncomfortable in arriving at a final diagnosis.

We as pediatricians have an additional advantage of approaching the child based on well-defined clinical symptoms which may suggest limited differential diagnosis and also taking the child's age into consideration, diagnostic possibility may be best explored and our vision may be narrowed down sharply towards better radiological diagnosis.

We have carefully concentrated more on the conventional, day-to-day method of basic radiological approach and restricted our approach to the unfamiliar imaging techniques.

In a true practical sense, the images given and the approaches aimed will be most useful to all of the pediatricians especially in the Indian context of restrained financial background and thus burden of investigation may not be much felt by the parents of sick children.

We have carefully dealt with the most of the acute conditions which are commonly seen in our outpatient clinic, pediatric casualty, PICU, NICU and in our day-to-day chamber practice.

We, the contributors will feel extremely happy if you are able to make a valid diagnosis after going through book and that ray of hope when radiated from you will be the day of success for this book.

The Editorial Team

Acknowledgments

With deep gratitude we acknowledge the Past National President of IAP Dr TU Sukumaran who whole heartedly supported and encouraged us to come out with a book in Basic classical X-rays in pediatrics. We are also very much pleased to acknowledge the current National President Dr Digant D Shastri for his encouragement extended to go for Second edition of this book. We very much appreciate all the editors of various chapters of this book, Dr Mona D Shastri, Dr G Vijayalakshmi, Dr Anoop Verma, Dr M Zulfikar Ahamed, Dr Anand Vasudev, Dr TK Nandakumaran, Dr Manish Kumar, Dr Kavita Menghani, and Dr Pulak Parag who have contributed much to revise this edition to the level of current requirement.

TM Ananda Kesavan
S Venkateswaran

Contents

Abbreviations

ACHD	Acyanotic Congenital Heart Disease	HMD	Hyaline Membrane Disease
AHD	Acquired Heart Disease	IDPA	Idiopathic Dilatation of Pulmonary Artery
ALCAPA	Anomalies Left Coronary Artery from Pulmonary Artery	IVC	Inferior Vena Cava
		LA	Left Atrium
		LAE	Left Atrial Enlargement
AP	Anteroposterior	LPA	Left Pulmonary Artery
AP Window	Aortopulmonary Window	L-TGA	L-Transposition of Great Arteries
AR	Aortic Regurgitation		
AS	Aortic Stenosis	LV	Left Ventricle
ASD	Atrial Septal Defect	MAPCA	Major Aortopulmonary Collateral Arteries
AVSD	Atrioventricular Septal Defect		
		MPA	Main Pulmonary Artery
BT Shunt	Blalock Taussig Shunt	MR	Mitral Regurgitation
CCHD	Congenital Cyanotic Heart Disease	MRI	Magnetic Resonance Imaging
CDH	Congenital Diaphragmatic Hernia	MS	Mitral Stenosis
		PA	Posteroanterior
CHD	Congenital Heart Disease	PAH	Pulmonary Arterial Hypertension
CoA	Coarctation of Aorta		
CR	Computerized Radiograph	PAWP	Pulmonary Artery Wedge Pressure
CTR	Cardiothoracic Ratio		
DCM	Dilated Cardiomyopathy	PBF	Pulmonary Blood Flow
DILV	Double Inlet Left Ventricle	PDA	Patent Ductus Arteriosus
DORV	Double Outlet Right Ventricle	PEM	Protein Energy Malnutrition
		PR	Pulmonary Regurgitation
DR	Digital Radiograph	PS	Pulmonary Stenosis
d-TGA	d-Transportation of Great Arteries	PV	Pulmonary Vein
		PVH	Pulmonary Venous Hypertension
HAPVC	Hemi Anomalous Pulmonary Venous Connection		
		PVOD	Pulmonary Vascular Occlusive Disease
HLHS	Hypoplastic Left Heart Syndrome	RA	Right Atrium
		RAE	Right Atrial Enlargement

RDPA	Right Descending Pulmonary Artery	RVOT	Right Ventricular Outflow Tract
RPA	Right Pulmonary Artery	SVC	Superior Vena Cava
RUPA	Right Upper Pulmonary Artery	TA	Tricuspid Atresia
RV	Right Ventricle	TAPVC	Total Anomalous Pulmonary Vein Connection
RV EMF	RV Endomyocardial Fibrosis	TOF	Tetralogy of Fallot
RVH	Right Ventricular Hypertrophy	VSD	Ventricular Septal Defect

Introduction

X-rays are most commonly used radiological investigation all over the world. Most of us are very familiar with chest X-rays (for many people X-ray means X-ray of chest!), because we can interpret it easily, freely available, cheap, and one can repeat it. The only disadvantage is the risk of radiation.

X-rays were discovered way back in 1825 and even now its use has not dimmed. X-rays are electromagnetic radiations. They are produced in a cathode ray tube where fast moving electrons from a filament strike a tungsten anode and the energy is converted into X-rays. When X-rays pass through the body they are absorbed to varying amounts, bone absorbing the most. The X-rays that exit the body are made to form an image on X-ray film, on an activated cassette (computerized radiography) or is directly digitized and is viewed on a computer (digital radiography). The image obtained of the body shows the internal body structures in white, black and shades of gray. Air is black in color as it is least dense, has not absorbed any radiation, and allows the X-rays to pass through easily. Bone and metal are white as they are very dense. Soft tissues like liver and spleen and fluid that may accumulate in the pleural cavity appear white, but not as densely white as bone.

Fluoroscopy using an image intensifier allows real-time imaging using X-rays. In this, the image is intensified and put on a TV monitor. This imaging is useful when motion in internal organs needs to be studied, e.g. respiratory motion in obstructive emphysema. Since radiation dose is high in this, intermittent rather than constant radiation exposure is used.

Fluoroscopy is also used for contrast studies. In this, an opaque medium like barium is used to line and fill hollow internal viscera. Barium is very dense and absorbs X-rays, thus appearing white. Barium can be ingested in Barium swallow and meal or can be instilled into the rectum and colon for a barium enema study. Air is also used as a contrast medium as in double contrast enema for rectal and colonic polyps. Barium enema is given, then evacuated and air is instilled into the colon under fluoroscopic guidance. This clearly brings out barium-coated white mucosal lesions against the black background of air.

Angiography is the study of blood vessels. The contrast media used here are iodine compounds. A peripheral artery is catheterized and contrast is injected into the required branches. Images are timed and taken rapidly and fine vascular detail is obtained in the X-rays. Computerized tomography of blood vessels uses contrast medium, but without invasive catheterization. In magnetic resonance angiography, blood vessels can be studied even without contrast, by computer manipulation.

The quest for better images and more precise diagnoses has led to rapid advancements in the field of radiology. The wide spectrum of modalities that are available in present times, enable us to study the morphology and function of the human body in explicit detail. However, in children almost 75% of questions arising from clinical problems are solved by X-rays and ultrasound. Even when other techniques are used, the X-ray usually serves as guidance to the choice of the next investigative modality (e.g. mediastinal masses discovered in chest X-ray is followed by CT). So X-rays need to be interpreted correctly. This book focusing only on X-ray radiography is a sincere effort aimed at sharpening the X-ray reading skills that will help in solving the majority of daily clinical problems.

It may be felt that imaging is now playing a large part in clinical diagnosis and that final diagnoses are obtained from imaging. While this may be true to a certain extent it should be remembered that clinical history and examination is the base and images have to be interpreted on the basis of clinical findings. Sharpening X-ray interpretation skills will help in mastering the use of the primary investigative modality that will help in diagnostic evaluation and treatment, ultimately for the benefit of the patient.

X-ray Imaging in Children

Mona D Shastri

■ INTRODUCTION

Radio imaging examinations are noninvasive tests that produce images of inside patient's body and provide valuable information to help diagnosis of illnesses and injuries.

The ray of hope for radiological investigation has first appeared on November 8, 1895, when physicist Professor Conrad Wilhelm Röntgen (1845–1923) stumbled on X-rays while experimenting with Lenard tubes and Crookes tubes and began studying them. He wrote an initial report "ON A NEW KIND OF RAY: A PRELIMINARY COMMUNICATION" and on December 28, 1895 submitted it to Würzburg's Physical-Medical Society journal. This was the first paper written on X-rays. Röntgen referred to the radiation as "X", to indicate that it was an unknown type of radiation. The name stuck, although (over Röntgen's great objections) many of his colleagues suggested calling them Röntgen rays. They are still referred to as such in many languages, including German, Hungarian, Danish, Polish, Swedish, Finnish, Estonian, Russian, Japanese, Dutch, Georgian, Hebrew, and Norwegian. Röntgen received the first Nobel Prize in Physics for his discovery.

X-rays are electromagnetic energy waves that act similarly to light rays, but at wave lengths approximately 1,000 times shorter than those of light. Röntgen holed up in his laboratory and conducted a series of experiments to better understand his discovery. He learned that X-rays penetrate human flesh but not higher-density substances such as bone or lead and that they can be photographed. He discovered their medical use when he made a picture of his wife's hand on a photographic plate formed due to X-rays. The photograph of his wife's hand was the first photograph of a human body part using X-rays. When she saw the picture, she said "I have seen my death". Röntgen immediately noticed X-rays could have medical applications. Along with his 28 December Physical-Medical Society submission he sent a letter to physicians he knew around Europe (January 1, 1896). The first use of X-rays under clinical conditions was by John Hall-Edwards in Birmingham, England on 11 January 1896, when he radiographed a needle stuck in the hand of an associate. On February 14, 1896 Hall-Edwards was also the first to use X-rays in a surgical operation.

Röntgen's discovery was labeled as medical miracle and X-rays soon became an important diagnostic tool in medicine, allowing doctors to see inside the human body for the first time without surgery. In 1897, X-rays were first used on a military battlefield, during the Balkan War, to find bullets and broken bones inside patients.

What is X-ray?

- ❏ X-rays are a form of electromagnetic waves that can penetrate through the body and the images appear in shades of black and white, depending on the type of tissue the X-rays pass through.
- ❏ Bones absorb more radiation and appear white on X-rays.
- ❏ Muscle or fat absorbs less, and appears in shades of gray on X-ray film.
- ❏ Air absorbs little of the X-rays, so the lungs appear black on an X-ray film.

■ TYPES OF X-RAYS

Conventional Plain X-rays

The most common of X-rays and is the cheapest modality of radiological investigation.

Computed Tomography (CT) Scans

Computer-based three-dimensional X-ray images are processed to create detailed pictures (scans) of cross-sections of the body.

Fluoroscopy

It is X-rays and a fluorescent screen to study moving or real-time structures in the body. When it is combined with swallowed or injected contrast agents the digestive processes or blood flow can be viewed. Clogged arteries can be opened by internally threaded contrast injected guided catheter using a fluoroscopy called cardiac angioplasty. Epidural injections or joint aspirations can be precisely done with the help of fluoroscopy.

▌ WHAT ARE THE DANGERS AND RISKS OF X-RAYS?

Radiation Hazards

When X-ray was first introduced, scientists were quick to realize the benefits of X-rays, but slower to comprehend the harmful effects of radiation. Initially, it was believed X-rays passed through flesh as harmlessly as light. However, within several years, researchers began to report cases of burns and skin damage after exposure to X-rays, and in 1904, Thomas Edison's assistant, Clarence Dally, who had worked extensively with X-rays, died of skin cancer. With the widespread experimentation with X-rays after their discovery in 1895 by scientists, physicians, and inventors came many stories of burns, hair loss, and worse in technical journals of the time. In February 1896, Professor John Daniel and Dr William Lofland Dudley of Vanderbilt University reported hair loss after Dr Dudley was X-rayed. A child who had been shot in the head was brought to the Vanderbilt laboratory in 1896. Daniel reported that 21 days after taking a picture of Dudley's skull (with an exposure time of 1 hour), he noticed a bald spot of 2 inches (5.1 cm) in diameter on the part of his head nearest the X-ray tube.

In August 1896 Dr HD Hawks, a graduate of Columbia College, suffered severe hand and chest burns from an X-ray demonstration. Elihu Thomson deliberately exposed a finger to an X-ray tube over a period of time and suffered pain, swelling, and blistering. Dally's death caused some scientists to begin taking the risks of radiation more seriously, but they still were not fully understood.

Though the risk of tissue damage due to X-ray radiation is relatively small, it may increase with cumulative repeated multiple X-ray exposure over one's life time. The risk of developing cancer, cataracts, and skin burns are likely to occur with cumulative exposure. Radiation does have some risks to consider, but it is also important to remember X-rays can help detect disease or injury at early stages so the ailment can be treated appropriately. Sometimes X-ray testing can be lifesaving.

BARIUM STUDIES FOR DIGESTIVE TRACT

Types of Barium X-rays

- Barium swallow
- Barium small bowel follow through
- Barium enema.

Barium Swallow

A barium swallow is to examine the back of the throat, esophagus, and stomach. With a barium swallow, the patient is asked to drink barium-containing chalky liquid. The indications for barium swallow include:

- Dysphagia
- Abdominal pain
- Unusual bloating
- Unexplained vomiting
- Weight loss of unexplained origin.

The barium coats the walls of the esophagus and stomach, which is then visible on X-rays. The test is effective in locating strictures, ulcers, hiatal hernias, erosions in the esophagus or stomach, muscle disorders such as achalasia, and other abnormalities such as esophageal cancer.

Barium Small Bowel Follow Through

Barium studies may also be used to look further down into the digestive tract. In a barium small bowel follow through the patient is observed as the barium passes beyond the stomach into the small intestine, and eventually makes its way to colon. In the procedure, the patient is often turned side to side to best visualize the small bowel or small intestine. A barium small bowel follow through may be done to help diagnose tumors of the small bowel, a small bowel obstruction, or inflammatory diseases of the small intestine such as Crohn's disease.

Indications

- Pain abdomen
- Rectal bleeding
- Unexplained vomiting
- Abnormal bowel movements
- Chronic diarrhea or constipation
- Dysphagia
- Unexplained weight loss
- Unusual bloating
- To locate anatomical abnormalities.

Barium Enema

It is modality of choice for detecting pathology of large bowel and ano rectal region. It is mainly used for Hirschsprung disease to detect length of aganglionic segment. Before the availability of ultrasound scanning it was modality to diagnose and treat large bowel (Colo-colic) intussusception. Pre-procedure bowel preparation is not required

RADIOGRAPHIC POSITIONINGS

- *Anterior*: Toward the front of the body
- *Posterior*: Toward the back of the body
- *Superior*: Toward the top of the body
- *Inferior*: Toward the bottom of the body
- *Medial*: Toward the midline
- *Lateral*: Away from the midline.

Body Positions

- Erect: Standing or sitting
- Decubitus: Lying down
- Supine: Lying on back
- Prone: Lying face-down
- Lateral decubitus: Lying on one side
  - Right lateral: Right side touches the cassette
  - Left lateral: Left side touches the cassette.

Views in Chest Radiography

- Posteroanterior (PA)
- Anteroposterior (AP) erect
- Supine
- Lateral
- Cross table lateral.

CHEST RADIOGRAPH

The *chest radiograph* is the most commonly requested radiographic examinations in the assessment of the *pediatric patient*.

Indications

- Respiratory distress
- Cardiac disease
- Bronchiolitis
- Pneumonia
- Pulmonary tuberculosis
- Pneumothorax
- Trauma
- Foreign bodies
- Line placement location (e.g. Endotracheal tube).

Projections

Regular Projections

- PA erect
- AP erect
- AP supine

Special Projections

- Lateral view and cross table lateral view
- To highlight pathology in the mediastinum, costophrenic recess and localize lesions.

Tips for Pediatric Chest Radiography

The challenges in acquiring radiographs in children are:
- Difficulty in achieving inspiration
- Likelihood of motion blurring
- Wide range of tissue densities
- Need to minimize radiation dose.

To overcome these:
- Attention diversion with toys, games, and/or conversation
- Immobilization with blankets and velcro straps
- Child-appropriate language.

IMPORTANCE OF DECUBITUS POSITION

Decubitus position: A position used in producing a radiograph of the chest or abdomen of a patient who is lying down, with the central ray horizontal.

The patient may be:
- Prone (ventral *decubitus*)
- Supine (dorsal *decubitus*)
- Left or right side (left or right lateral *decubitus*).
- *Lateral decubitus view of the chest*: To demonstrate small pleural effusions, pneumothorax, and inhaled foreign bodies.

Image Evaluation

- Side marking should be clearly labeled.
- In an ideal chest X-ray, lung fields should be visible from the apices down to the lateral costophrenic angles
- No superimposition of chin over any structures
- No superimposition of the scapulae borders on the lung fields
- Sternoclavicular joints at equidistance
- Clavicle should be in the same horizontal plane
- A minimum of nine posterior ribs should be visualized above the diaphragm
- Ribs and thoracic cage are seen only faintly over the heart
- Clearly visible vascular markings of the lungs.

Lateral Decubitus for Pleural Effusions

The fluid in the chest gets layered when the patient lies on the suspected side and can be viewed by chest X-ray in the lateral decubitus position is more sensitive and can detect as little as 50 mL of fluid. At least 300 mL of fluid must be present before upright chest X-rays can detect a pleural effusion.

Respiratory System

S Venkateswaran

CHEST

Know the normal chest X-ray first?

A good pediatrician must be able to recognize normal roentgenographic chest before attempting to explore the radiopathology. It is more of identifying the normal shape, contour, and densities of visualized structures in the chest. It is mainly comparing the whiteness and darkness of one half with that of other half.

Chest posteroanterior (PA) view: The norms to be observed.

Whether the film is taken with the required norms?

- ❏ Whether it is anteroposterior (AP) or PA view?
- ❏ Whether it is taken in deep (full) inspiration or expiration?
- ❏ Whether positioning is correct or tilted?
- ❏ Whether side marking is given?
- ❏ Whether all required anatomic parts are included in the film?

How to Differentiate between AP and PA Film of the Chest?

In AP view (Fig. 2.1):
- ❏ The lung volume is reduced
- ❏ The lung appears rectangular because of horizontally placed diaphragmatic leaflet and inwardly placed scapular margin

- ❏ The heart appears increased in size because of elevated diaphragm
- ❏ The costophrenic and cardiophrenic angles give false appearance of pleural effusion.

In PA view (Fig. 2.2):
- ❏ The anatomical shape of the lung is visualized
- ❏ Well aerated clear lungs are seen
- ❏ Lateral chest wall margin is well delineated
- ❏ Diaphragmatic leaflets with its normal curvature is well distinguished
- ❏ Costophrenic and cardiophrenic angles are clearly seen.

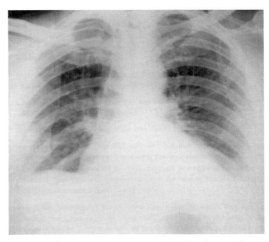

Fig. 2.1: Chest anteroposterior view. The lung volume appears to be reduced and the heart appears to be increased in size, which are all because of inwardly turned scapulae and elevated diaphragm.

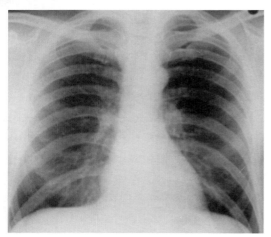

Fig. 2.2: Chest posteroanterior view. The entire area of the lung and all the margins including the diaphragmatic leaflets are well delineated.

How to Order for a Chest X-ray?

☐ Order by chief complaint
☐ Order the correct view
☐ *Posteroanterior view*: Standard frontal chest film
☐ *Lateral view*: Marked by which side of chest is against the film
☐ Order the correct position:
  • Lying vs. upright
  • Right vs. left.

What is to be Observed before Interpreting a Film?

☐ Make sure it is the right patient
☐ Know the patient's detail
☐ Have older films if available
☐ Place the film on the view box as though you are facing the patient.

Go for Systematic Interpretation

Suggested routines:
Look for label and other data base:

1. *Name*: Since the names can be shared by others, check for the hospital number if any.

2. *Date*: Important for comparing prior exams. Serial images to be numbered.
3. *Position markers*: Right (Rt) vs. Left (Lt)
4. *Position of the patient*:
  • AP
  • AP supine
  • PA view
  • Lateral (Lt/Rt) for anatomy reading
  • Lordotic view for apical region
  • Lateral decubitus (Lt/Rt) for effusion or thickening
  • Oblique (Rt/Lt; posterior/anterior): eliminate superimposed lesion.
5. *Quality of the film*: One should be able to see the outlines of the vertebral bodies within the heart shadow.
6. *Rotation*: Should be minimal. It can be assessed by comparing the medial ends of clavicle to the margins of vertebral body at the same level. This should be at equidistance on either side.

Systematic Interpretation

Systematic interpretation is done with a search for pathology.

Reading a chest X-ray requires systematic approach. It is tempting to leap to the obvious findings but failure to be systematic can lead to missing pathologies, overlooking more subtle lesions, drawing false conclusions, based on a film that is technically poor. This may lead on to wrong management on an inaccurate interpretation.

The best way of learning how to spot abnormalities on a chest X-ray is to look lot of them repeatedly both normal and abnormal. This reduces the chances of missing and difficult to see features.

General Principles

☐ Read X-ray yourself
☐ Be systematic

- ❏ Be aware of common artifacts
- ❏ Serially compare
- ❏ Observe symmetry
- ❏ Believe you missed a finding until you confirm that your review is clear.

Reading Order of a Chest X-ray

One of the commonly used methods is given below:

- ❏ General review
- ❏ Centering of the film
- ❏ Trachea
- ❏ Mediastinum
- ❏ Hilum
- ❏ Diaphragm
- ❏ Heart
- ❏ Lung
- ❏ Soft tissues, skeleton, and artifacts.

Pathological Search

1. General review:
   Is the film well penetrated and symmetrical?
2. Centering of the film:
   Is the image centered?—Inner clavicular ends should be at the same distance from the midline.
3. Trachea:
   Is the trachea central?
   Rotation is the most common cause for inequality in the translucency of the lungs and needs to be differentiated from increased transradiancy from other causes.
4. Mediastinum:
   Are there any bumps that should not be there?
   What might they be?
   - Masses
   - Lymph nodes
   - Thymus
   - Thymoma.

5. Hilum:
   How is the hila?
   - Normal relationship
   - Size.
6. Diaphragm:
   - Does the lowest part of the heart shadow meet the diaphragm at a sharply defined angle? If not why?
   - Does the dome of the diaphragm have a normal sweep? If not why?
   - Does the outer edge of the diaphragm meet the pleura at a sharp acute angle? If not why?
   - Look for any pathological variations in relation to diaphragm
     » Air under diaphragm
     » Flattened diaphragm
     » Loss of diaphragm definition
     » Elevated hemidiaphragm
     » Tenting of diaphragm.
7. Heart:
   - *Right border*: Edge of right atrium
   - *Left border*: (L) ventricle + (L) atrium
   - *Anterior border*: Right ventricle
   - *Posterior border*: Left ventricle—assess for the size, shape, and position of the heart and pulmonary circulation.

   The cardiothoracic ratio (CT ratio) is usually about 50% but can be more in the first year of life and a large thymus can make assessment difficult as with a film in poor inspiration. As with adults, one-third should be to the right of center and two-thirds to the left.

   Assessment of pulmonary circulation can be important in congenital heart disease but can be very difficult in routine practice. Heart appears water dense seen usually with the apex to the left, occupies about 50% of chest width at widest point. Aortic knob may be seen through thymus on left.

   Pulmonary vessels can be seen in hila, best on lateral view. The vessels are seen extending to midlung tapering gradually.

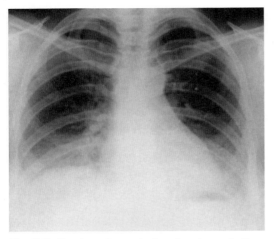 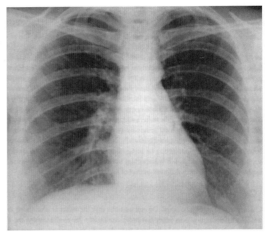

Fig. 2.3: Chest posteroanterior view in expiration. Because of the elevated diaphragm in expiration the lung volume appears reduced with a pseudo appearance of bilateral basal congestion and enlarged heart.

Fig. 2.4: Chest posteroanterior view in full inspiration. Fully expanded lung showing maximum lung volume, clear outlines, and well delineated diaphragmatic leaflets.

8. Lungs:
   - *Assess the lung volume*: Count down the anterior rib ends to the one that meets the middle of the hemidiaphragm. A good inspirating film should have the anterior end of the 5th or 6th rib meeting the middle of the diaphragm. More than six anterior ribs show hyperinflation. Fewer than five indicates an expiratory film or under inflation. With under inflation as in expiratory film, the third or fourth rib crosses the diaphragm. This makes normal lungs appear opaque and a normal heart appears enlarged (Figs. 2.3 and 2.4).
   - *Lung density*: Lungs are uniformly aerated and they appear black on most films. Divide the lungs arbitrarily into upper, middle, and lower zones and compare the two sides for size and density.
   Evaluate pulmonary vascular pattern and compare the upper to lower lobe, right to left, normal tapering to periphery.
   - *Pleura*: Follow the pleura around the rib cage. Look for major and minor fissures if seen. Compare the hemidiaphragms, which must curve downward and that the costophrenic and cardiophrenic angles should be sharp and clear and not blunted.

9. Soft tissues, skeleton, and artifacts:
   - Breast shadow especially in an adolescent girl may show slightly increased density and look for symmetrical shadows.
   - Look for scapula, humerus, shoulder joint, clavicle, and ribs for their symmetry. Review spine and rib cage for alignment, disk space narrowing, lytic and blastic regions, etc.
   - Recognize the artifacts such as skin folds which may mimic pneumothorax. In girls, either plaited or dressed with ornaments may cause a variety of artifacts usually projected over the upper lobe and mediastinum.

10. The other ways of looking into the chest A – B – C – D – E – F – G – H approach to interpretation of chest X-ray.

A: Airway
B: Bone
C: Cardiovascular
D: Diaphragm
E: Extrapulmonary
F: Lung Field
G: Gastric bubble
H: Hilum.

How a normal chest should look like?

The basic principle in AP or PA view is a matter of comparing the shape and densities of the various structures visualized (Fig. 2.5).

☐ Both lungs should have equal but relatively darker density because of aeration

☐ Heart as a whole should have uniform density of opaqueness, as it is due to water density

☐ Both hilar regions should be of relatively equal density

☐ Cardiac silhouette to either side of the spine should be of about the same density

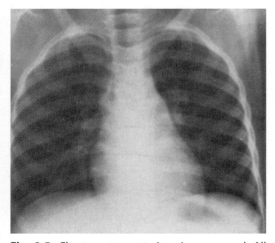

Fig. 2.5: Chest posteroanterior view—normal. All regions and borders, lung volume on either side, both hilar regions and both diaphragmatic leaflets appear normal.

☐ The juxtapositioned margins of the heart and diaphragmatic leaflet in a normally aerated lung should be crisp and distinct.

Lateral view:

☐ Identify the sternum anteriorly and spine posteriorly

☐ Divide the space vertically as retrocardiac and retrosternal

☐ In retrosternal space, the superior half is always radiolucent because of normally aerated upper lobe of the lung

☐ Rarely in infancy, due to normal thymus the radiolucency is replaced by radio-density or whiteness

☐ The retrosternal lower half is opaque due to cardiac shadow

☐ The retrocardiac superoposterior region is relatively opaque than the lower half due to the soft tissues of the upper chest wall, axillae, and shoulder.

☐ The lower half of retrocardiac space is characteristically radiolucent due to normally aerated superimposed lower lobe.

The two important characters of right diaphragmatic leaflet are (Figs. 2.6 and 2.7):

1. Its position is slightly higher than the left
2. Usually seen in its entirety, right up to its insertion on to the anterior chest wall.

The third but rare character of right diaphragmatic leaflet is that inferior vena cava being right-sided blends with the right diaphragmatic leaflet.

The characteristic features of the left diaphragmatic leaflet are (Fig. 2.8):

1. Its level is little lower than that of right
2. Usually is seen up to the posterior cardiac wall and at this point it blends with the cardiac silhouette
3. The gastric bubble mostly lies under this leaflet.

Note: All of these findings and relationships may not be evident in every lateral chest film, but enough of them are usually present.

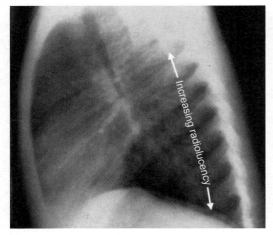

Fig. 2.6: Chest lateral view. Lateral view showing increasing radiolucency from top to bottom of the retrocardiac space.

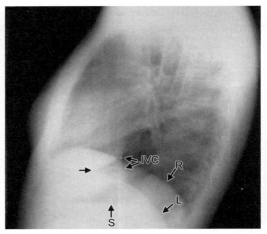

Fig. 2.8: Localization of the diaphragmatic leaflet. The right diaphragmatic leaflet is higher than the left and is seen in its entirety while the left one blends with the posterior aspect of the cardiac silhouette.

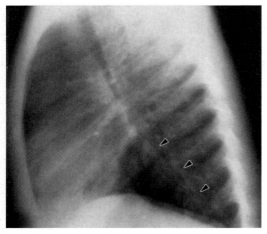

Fig. 2.7: Chest lateral view. Normal lower lobe pulmonary vessels mimicking pulmonary infiltrate.

PNEUMONIAS

The Viral Spectrum

Any viral infection of the lower respiratory tract can produce roentgenographically patterns ranging from the infiltrate free lungs of bronchiolitis to the diffusely infiltrated lungs seen with widespread parenchymal pneumonitis. Any one of these or of the entire spectrum is demonstrable especially during viral epidemic. Most of the viral infection being tracheobronchial in nature the predominant feature is that of "parahilar peribronchial infiltrate".

The important pathological changes that occur in viral respiratory infections are:

☐ Tracheobronchial inflammation, the inflammatory thickening, and edema of bronchial and peribronchial predisposes to airway narrowing with tendency for air trapping and parahilar infiltrate (Fig. 2.9).

☐ In the one end of the spectrum of viral lower respiratory tract infection (LRTI) is the young infant with bronchiolitis and the incidence peaks around 6 months, but it is common up to 2 years of age or so. It may roentgenographically appear as overaeration and in three types of form.

Bronchiolitis with Relatively Clear Lungs

Posteroanterior view (Fig. 2.10):

☐ Considerable overaeration
☐ Complete absence of peripheral infiltrates
☐ Minimal parahilar infiltrate.

Lateral view (Fig. 2.11):
- ❏ Marked overaeration
- ❏ Characteristically bell-shaped chest
- ❏ Markedly depressed and flattened diaphragmatic leaflets.

Bronchiolitis with Parahilar, Peribronchial Infiltrate

Posteroanterior view:
- ❏ Marked overaeration of both lungs
- ❏ Some parahilar peribronchial infiltrate (Fig. 2.12).

Lateral view (Fig. 2.13):
- ❏ Marked depression and flattening of the diaphragmatic leaflet, secondary to overaeration
- ❏ In the upper retrosternal area thymus gland is separated from heart due to overaeration.

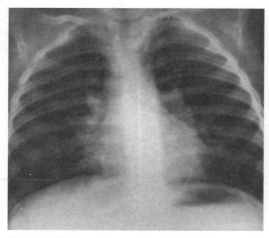

Fig. 2.9: Viral parahilar peribronchial infiltrate with adenopathy.

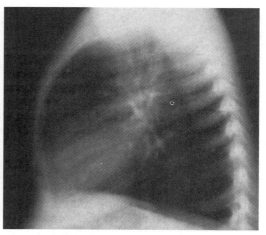

Fig. 2.11: Bronchiolitis, lateral view. Classic bell-shaped chest due to overaeration.

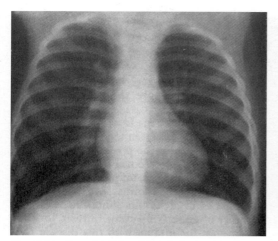

Fig. 2.10: Bronchiolitis with relatively clear lungs. Hyperaerated hyperlucent lung.

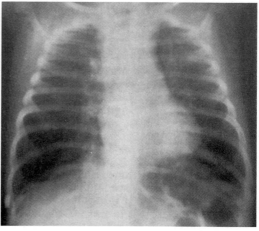

Fig. 2.12: Bronchiolitis with parahilar peribronchial infiltrate.

Viral LRTI with Atelectasis Mimicking Pneumonia

Segmental atelectasis, single or multiple, unilateral or bilateral, because of combined effect of mucosal inflammation, endobronchial secretions, and mucus plugs may result in bronchial obstruction and may have a propensity to mimic pneumonia. But a clue for viral diagnosis, due to rapid clearing of respiratory distress symptoms usually in less than 24 hours could be kept in mind, as it is often due to rapid dislodging of mucus plug.

This child presented with acute onset of fever of 102°F, marked respiratory distress, and mild cyanosis.

Overaeration: There is generalized overaeration:
- ❑ Peribronchial infiltrate (Fig. 2.14)
- ❑ Patchy consolidation at right lower lobe.

Next day:
- ❑ Pneumonic patch disappeared
- ❑ Peribronchial infiltrate persists (Fig. 2.15).
- ❑ Such a rapid clearing is not possible with bacterial pneumonia.

Hilar adenopathy: A varying degrees of hilar adenopathy from nil to well-circumscribed lymph node, further accentuating the parahilar density (Figs. 2.16 and 2.17).

Pneumonitis: Inflammatory extension and mucus exudation may cause either alveolar or interstitial pneumonitis (Fig. 2.18).

The interstitial pattern is characterized by streaky or reticular infiltrate coursing through the lungs or radiating from the prominent hilar regions into the parenchyma presenting at times typically as "shaggy heart" appearance (Fig. 2.19). Alveolar infiltrate can be nodular, fluffy, patchy or consolidative and at times it may be difficult to differentiate from similar infiltrates produced by bacterial infections (Fig. 2.20). These patients in spite of obvious roentgenographic patterns are clinically less ill.

There may be even gross discrepancy between the patients' clinical condition and the X-ray findings (Fig. 2.21).

Posteroanterior view:
- ❑ Fluffy, ill-defined parenchymal infiltrate in the right and left upper lobes.

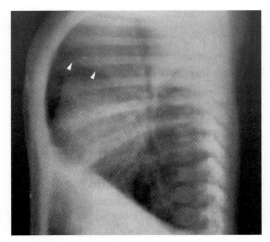

Fig. 2.13: Lateral view in a bronchiolitis. Overaeration depressing the diaphragmatic leaflets and lifting the thymus.

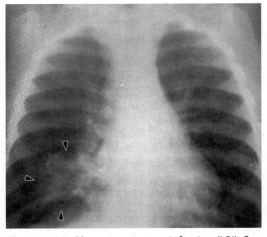

Fig. 2.14: Viral lower respiratory infection (LRI), first admission day picture. Viral LRI with atelectasis mimicking pneumonia.

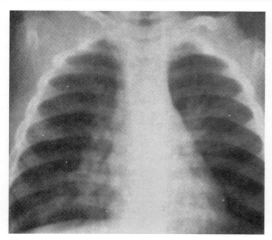

Fig. 2.15: Viral LRI, second admission day picture. Fastest resolution of lower lobe lesion is possibly of resolving atelectasis following mucus plug dislodging.

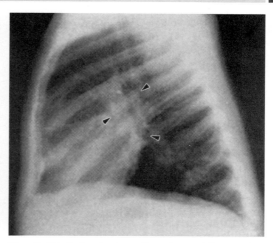

Fig. 2.17: Lateral view. Prominent hilar region partly due to adenopathy and partly due to peribronchial inflammation.

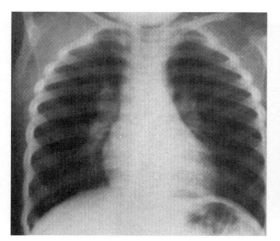

Fig. 2.16: Viral parahilar infiltrates and hilar adenopathy. Prominent hilar adenopathy with parahilar peribronchial infiltrate.

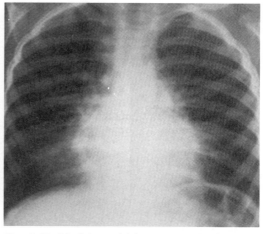

Fig. 2.18: Viral interstitial pneumonia. There are streaky infiltrates radiating from the parahilar region into the parenchyma of the lung giving the typical "shaggy heart" appearance.

❑ A consolidation in the right middle lobe.
❑ Round infiltrate in the right lower lobe behind the heart.

Atelectasis and obstructive emphysema: Thick, viscid, inflammatory mucus plugging may present with varying degrees of distal atelectasis.

Clinically

These children may present with cough, tachypnea, fever, coryza, and sinus congestion. The cough may be even croupy. On auscultation the findings could be either a transmitted upper airway sound or true rales,

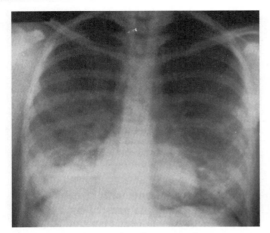

Fig. 2.19: Hazy lungs of viral interstitial pneumonitis. Diffuse haziness of the lungs and some reticulation in the lung bases.

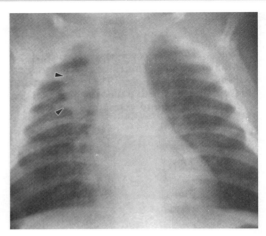

Fig. 2.21: Viral alveolar pneumonitis. Right upper lobe consolidation—a rare pattern of alveolar infiltration.

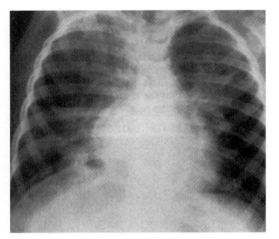

Fig. 2.20: Viral alveolar pneumonia. Bilateral ill-defined fluffy infiltrate in the upper lobes and consolidation in the right middle lobe and a round infiltrate in the right lower lobe behind the heart.

rhonchi and even wheezes can be heard. More commonly these sounds may change its character from time to time.

Obstructive Emphysema

When a major bronchus plugged by mucus, the entire lobe collapses or becomes emphysematous. This because of air trapping and the resultant hyperaeration is best seen during expiration, because the air will be emptied on the uninvolved side and the diaphragmatic leaflet will also be elevated on that side. But on the involved side air is trapped and diaphragm remains static or become flattened and the lung on that side appears hyperlucent.

Emphysema

This is another aeration disturbance commonly seen with LRTI especially with isolated lower lobe involvement. In such cases, the uninvolved and normal remaining lobe tends to be overaerated on inspiration and appears blacker.

Compensatory Emphysema

There is an infiltrate and partial atelectasis of the left lower lobe and because of this there is compensatory inspiratory overdistension and greater radiolucency of the left upper lobe (Fig. 2.22). Also note the level of right diaphragmatic leaflet.

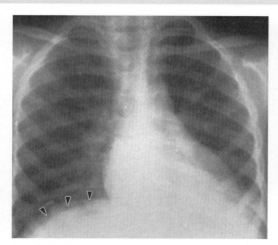

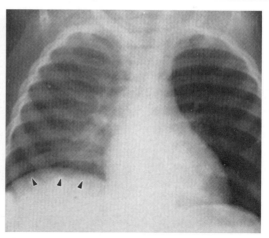

Fig. 2.22: Compensatory emphysema vs. obstructive emphysema. Compensatory emphysema of the left upper lobe with an infiltrate and partial atelectasis of the left lower lobe.

Fig. 2.23: Compensatory emphysema vs. obstructive emphysema. Obstructive emphysema of the left upper lobe in an expiratory film showing normal air expulsion in the right lung but trapped air in the left side.

Obstructive Emphysema

This film (Fig. 2.23) taken during expiration in which air is emptied from the right lung but on the left it is trapped in the left upper lobe. There is an infiltrate in the left lower lobe behind the left side of the heart.

The clinical note to realize in such situations is that these occurrences are temporary and that given enough time the findings will disappear.

Keynotes:

- ❐ Radiographic images of viral respiratory infections are of bizarre in nature
- ❐ Roentgenographically so called "parahilar peribronchial" infiltration results in prominent and "dirty parahilar regions"
- ❐ Interpretation of viral respiratory radiography at times is subjective and will vary from viewer to viewer
- ❐ Most of the viral respiratory chest images are temporary and are likely to be changing from time to time.

Bacterial Spectrum

Clinically, patients with bacterial pneumonias often present with abrupt onset of fever, lassitude, malaise, and cough with chest pain. As opposed to viral infections auscultatory localization of decreased air entry into involved area are usually clearly apparent in bacterial pneumonia.

Before interpreting bacterial pneumonias following practical aspects should be kept in mind for wide and variant approaches.

Clinically Evident Symptomatic Pneumonias with Normal Chest X-ray

The patient who obtains his/her chest roentgenograms early in the course of the disease, and because of the usual delay period of up to 12 hours from the onset of symptoms to the appearance of a roentgenographically demonstrable infiltrate the chest X-ray can be normal.

*Negative Auscultation with
Positive Chest Image*

It is important to note that it is not uncommon for auscultation to fail to detect a well-developed lobar pneumonia which turns out to be startlingly present roentgenographically. These cases represent instances of advanced consolidation and most likely breath sounds from the adjacent normal lung are so well transmitted through the consolidated lobe that it sounds normal on casual auscultation.

Subtle Pneumonia

Posteroanterior view: There is unilateral increase in density in the right apical region, which is likely to be missed as a normal soft tissue density (Fig. 2.24).

Lateral view: This view clearly demonstrates pneumonia in the posterior segment of the right upper lobe (Fig. 2.25).

Picking up Subtle Pneumonias

Early or minimal infiltrate are so subtle that they are totally overlooked or simply

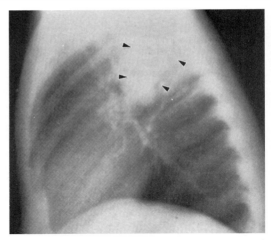

Fig. 2.25: Hiding right apical pneumonia. Lateral view brings out the pneumonia in the posterior segment of the right upper lobe.

misinterpreted as fortuitous conglomerations of rib and bronchovascular densities. The only way to diagnose such pneumonias is to be suspicious of and then methodically substantiate any focal area of increased density either by lateral chest film or by applying "Felson's silhouette sign".

Subtle Early Infiltrate

❑ There is a vague area of focal infiltration in the upper lung field lateral to the left hilar region (arrows) (Fig. 2.26).
❑ *Lateral view*: Substantiates the presence of this infiltrate as there is corresponding area of focally increased density in the posterior chest, superimposed over the spine (Fig. 2.27).

Lateral Chest Film

The value of the lateral chest views cannot be overstated in diagnosing early pneumonias. The usefulness of lateral view will be more evident and also one may be totally surprised at how well a pneumonia is visible

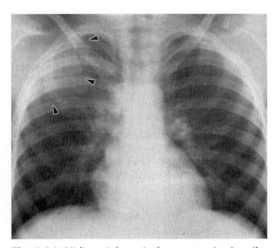

Fig. 2.24: Hiding right apical pneumonia. A unilateral increased focus of density over the right apex.

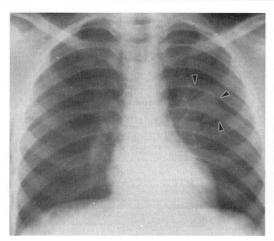

Fig. 2.26: Subtle early infiltrate. There is a vague area of focal infiltration in the left upper lung field, just lateral to the left hilar region.

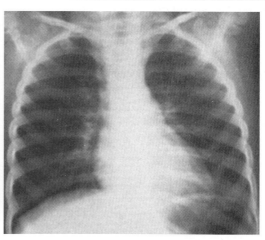

Fig. 2.28: Value of a lateral chest film. Only subtle indistinct left diaphragmatic leaflet and a little higher than normal.

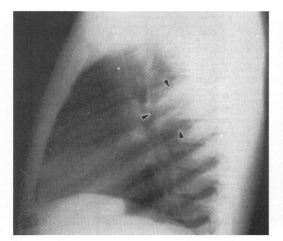

Fig. 2.27: Subtle early infiltrate. Lateral view brings out the focally increased density superimposed over the spine.

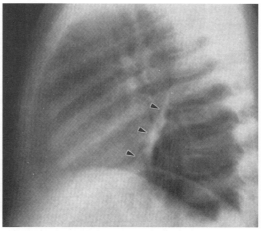

Fig. 2.29: Value of a lateral chest film. A clearly visualized left lower lobe pneumonia, just behind the left major fissure.

on the lateral view, and yet how poorly demarcated it is on the frontal projection. Never neglect to get a lateral view.

Value of the Lateral Chest Film

❏ The infiltrate is so subtle on this view which needs close inspection and one might note that the left diaphragmatic leaflet is slightly indistinct and slightly elevated due to secondary splinting (Fig. 2.28).

❏ *Lateral view*: Clearly bring out the left lower lobe pneumonia just behind the left major fissure (Fig. 2.29).

Applying Felson's Silhouette Sign

When two structures of equal roentgeno-graphic density are juxtaposed the interphase between them becomes obliterated. For example: The heart with a water density with aerated lung having air density which is normally juxtaposed, the cardiac edge is clearly demarcated.

But when the heart with water density is juxtaposed against another water density of pulmonary infiltrate then the interphase becomes indistinct or frankly obliterated and this is called "positive silhouette sign" due to adjacent pneumonic consolidation.

☐ Lower two-thirds of right cardiac border is indistinct and obliterated. The left cardiac border is sharp (Fig. 2.30).

☐ *Lateral view*: Confirms the presence of right middle lobe consolidation antero-inferiorly (Fig. 2.31).

Left Diaphragmatic Leaflet Silhouette Sign

☐ The clue to the suspicion is indistinct left diaphragmatic leaflet against the clearly visualized gastric air bubble (Fig. 2.32).

☐ Lateral view confirms the left lower lobe pneumonia posterior to the major fissure (Fig. 2.33).

☐ Positive silhouette sign in the right dia-phragm (Fig. 2.34).

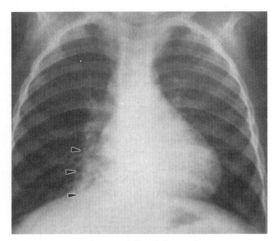

Fig. 2.30: Right middle lobe silhouette sign. Obliterated and indistinct right cardiac border by an adjacent pneumonia in the medial segment of right middle lobe.

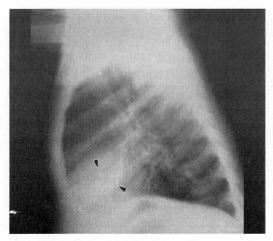

Fig. 2.31: Right middle lobe silhouette sign. Lateral view confirms the right middle lobe pneumonia.

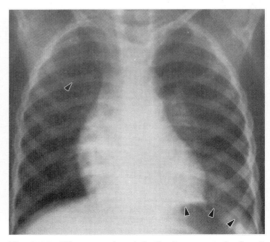

Fig. 2.32: Silhouette sign, left diaphragmatic leaflet. A strong clue for the presence of an infiltrate in the lower left lung field is indistinct left diaphragmatic leaflet.

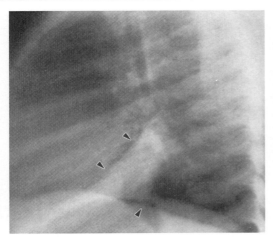

Fig. 2.33: Silhouette sign, left diaphragmatic leaflet. Lateral view confirms the left lower lobe pneumonia.

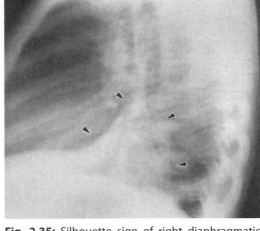

Fig. 2.35: Silhouette sign of right diaphragmatic leaflet. Lateral view confirms the right lower lobe pneumonia lying posterior to the major fissure.

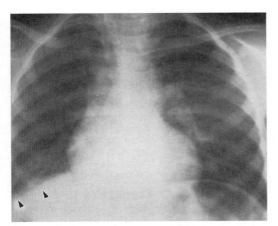

Fig. 2.34: Silhouette sign of right diaphragmatic leaflet. Positive silhouette sign of right diaphragm.

❏ Lateral view confirms right lower lobe pneumonia (Fig. 2.35).

Unfortunately, the silhouette sign also occurs under some normal situation. This normal variation occurs most often along the right cardiac border.

Normal Variation of Right Middle Lobe Silhouette Sign

Posteroanterior view: Poor inspiration and normal clustering of the bronchovascular markings adjacent to the right cardiac border causes obliteration of right heart border. This could be misinterpreted for a right middle lobe, medial segment, and pneumonia (Fig. 2.36).

Lateral view (Fig. 2.37): There is no infiltrate in the right middle lobe.

Pseudofocal Pneumonia

Due to right parahilar peribronchial infiltrate.

❏ The film taken in lordotic view, by virtue of the ribs appear horizontal posteriorly and slanted downward anteriorly. With the clustering of bronchovascular markings and parahilar peribronchial infiltrate with obliterated right heart border right middle lobe, medial segment pneumonia was suggested (Fig. 2.38).

❏ The lateral view rules out right middle lobe pneumonia (Fig. 2.39).

The reasons for such variations are:

❏ Blending of prominent bronchovascular markings with the right cardiac border

❏ Film taken in partial inspiration

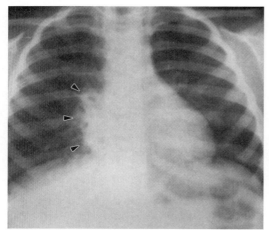

Fig. 2.36: Right middle lobe silhouette sign—normal variation. Normal clustering of broncho-vascular markings due to poor inspiration obliterating the cardiac silhouette, suggesting right middle lobe, medial segment pneumonia.

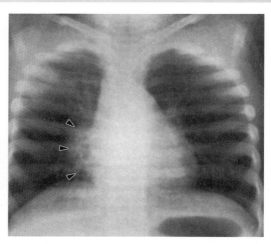

Fig. 2.38: Pseudofocal pneumonia. Hilar clustering of the right bronchovascular markings due to lordotic position of the chest film, suggesting right middle lobe medial segment pneumonia.

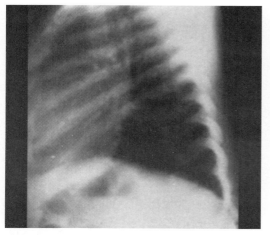

Fig. 2.37: Right middle lobe silhouette sign—normal variation. On lateral view there is no infiltrate in the right middle lobe.

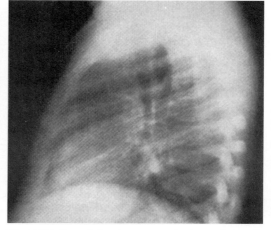

Fig. 2.39: Pseudofocal pneumonia. Lateral view is found to be normal and the posteroanterior view lesion is more of a positional default.

❏ When the film is obtained with the patient in partial lordotic position
❏ Merging of clustered bronchovascular markings with viral inflammatory parahilar peribronchial infiltrate with that of right cardiac border.

Looking for Hiding Pneumonias

There are certain areas which are notorious for hiding early pulmonary infiltrates. Unless one becomes thoroughly familiar with these hiding places, pulmonary infiltrate can be totally missed.

The favorite hiding places are:

- Behind the left side of the heart in the lower lobe extending into the costophrenic angle
- Behind the right side of the heart in the right lower lobe extending into costophrenic angle
- Behind the hilar regions in the superior segments of either lower lobe
- Deep in the posterior costophrenic sulcus behind the stomach, spleen or left lobe of liver
- High in the upper lobes
- Deep in the lateral costophrenic sulcus.

Hiding Left Lower Lobe Pneumonia, behind the Heart

- Vague area of increased density behind the left side of heart (arrowheads; Figs. 2.40 and 2.41).
- *Lateral view*: Pneumonia to be the left lower lobe deep in the costophrenic recess (arrowheads; Fig. 2.41).

Hiding Pneumonia behind the Right Side of the Heart

- Focal area of increased density behind the heart with the positive cardiac silhouette (Fig. 2.42).
- Confirmation of right lower lobe pneumonia behind the heart (Fig. 2.43).

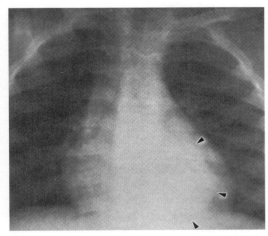

Fig. 2.40: Hiding left lower lobe pneumonia behind the heart. Large area of increased density behind the left side of the heart.

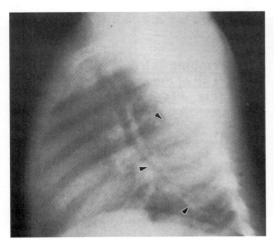

Fig. 2.41: Hiding left lower lobe pneumonia behind the heart. Lateral view showing the pneumonia in the left lower lobe.

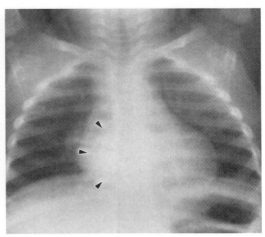

Fig. 2.42: Hiding pneumonia behind the right side of the heart. There is a focal area of increased density projected through the right side of the cardiac silhouette.

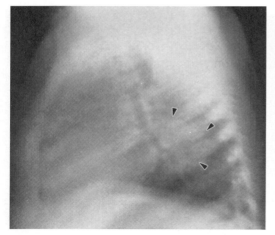

Fig. 2.43: Hiding pneumonia behind the right side of the heart. Lateral view confirms the presence of right lower lobe pneumonia.

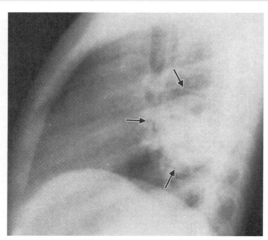

Fig. 2.45: Hiding pneumonia behind the left hilum. Lateral view shows the retrocarinal position of the superior segment of the left lobe pneumonia.

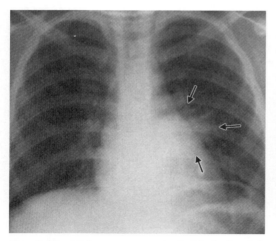

Fig. 2.44: Hiding pneumonia behind the left hilum. Denser and larger left hilum than the right.

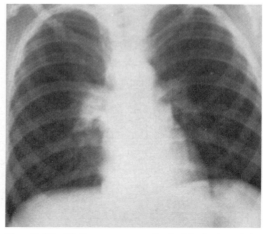

Fig. 2.46: Hiding pneumonia behind the right hilum. Large right hilum with increased density suggesting unilateral adenopathy.

Hiding Pneumonia behind the Left Hilum

☐ Left hilum is slightly denser and larger than the right (arrows; Fig. 2.44).

☐ *Lateral view:* Confirms the pneumonia to be in the superior segment of the left lower lobe (Fig. 2.45).

Hiding Pneumonia behind the Right Hilum

☐ Right hilum is slightly denser and larger than the left hilum (Fig. 2.46)

☐ Lateral view confirms the pneumonia to be in the superior segment of right lower lobe (Fig. 2.47).

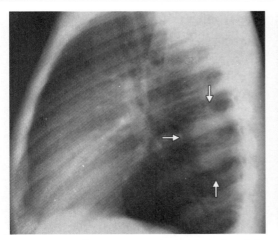

Fig. 2.47: Hiding pneumonia behind the right hilum. Lateral view showing the retrocarinal position of lesion to be due to superior segment pneumonia.

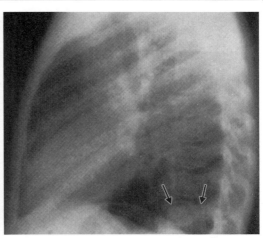

Fig. 2.49: Focal pneumonia, right lower lobe behind the liver. Lateral view showing the pneumonia lying deep in the posterior costophrenic sulcus.

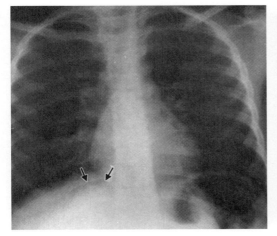

Fig. 2.48: Focal pneumonia, right lower lobe behind the liver. There is a focal area of increased density projected through the medial aspect of the liver silhouette.

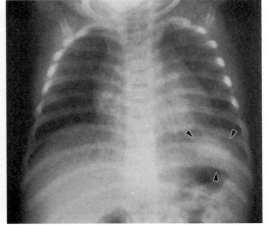

Fig. 2.50: Subtle focal pneumonia behind left diaphragmatic leaflet. A vague area of increased density projected through the left diaphragmatic leaflet, a consolidation of left lower lobe deep in the posterior costophrenic sulcus.

Hiding Pneumonia behind the Liver and Right Diaphragmatic Leaflet

☐ Focal area of opacification behind the medial aspect of liver silhouette (Fig. 2.48)
☐ Lateral view confirms it to be in deep position in the posterior costophrenic recess (Fig. 2.49).

Hiding Pneumonia behind the Left Diaphragmatic Leaflet

There is an area of increased density projected through the left diaphragmatic leaflet, lying in the posterior costophrenic sulcus (Fig. 2.50).

Miscellaneous Pneumonias

Though bilateral dense diffuse haziness are more often seen with viral pneumonias similar infiltrates can be seen with *Pneumocystis carinii* pneumonia, lipoid pneumonitis, and on chronicity in pulmonary hemosiderosis, the Hamman-Rich syndrome and pulmonary alveolar proteinosis.

Adenovirus infection when they prone to produce chronic lung damage may develop into Swyer-James lung.

Desquamative interstitial pneumonias are though rare in children, the picture may range from normally appearing lung with one of the lung showing parahilar peribronchial infiltrate to diffuse interstitial haziness or reticularity.

Varicella and infectious mononucleosis especially in adolescents that to in an immunologically suppressed child may present with primary pulmonary pneumonia. Mycoplasma pneumonia may present ranging from clearly looking acute lobar consolidation or diffuse nodular infiltrate and to any number of intervening roentgenographic patterns.

Bacterial pneumonias such as those due to *Staphylococcus aureus*, *Haemophilus influenzae* type B, and *Streptococcus pneumoniae* may at times be associated with empyema and pleural effusion.

When pneumonia occurring in sickle cell anemia we have to give importance to pneumococcal pneumonia, *Haemophilus influenzae* type B, and *Mycoplasma pneumoniae*.

Lobar consolidation in Friedlander's pneumonia may tend to expand the lobe and bulge the surrounding pictures outward.

Fungal infections of the lung are though rare in children, but may be so common in the so called fungus belt and the findings are so variable ranging from diffuse fluffy pulmonary infiltrate to those mimicking all forms of primary pulmonary tuberculosis.

Tuberculous Pneumonias

This being one of the most common problem, the most common confronted picture is that of unilateral hilar or paratracheal adenopathy. The other types of presentations are lobar or segmental consolidation, lobar or segmental atelectasis, lobar emphysema, pulmonary infiltration, and pleural effusion.

So, the rule of thumb for suspecting primary pulmonary tuberculosis is "unilateral hilar or paratracheal adenopathy alone, with or without parenchymal change of any type should be presumed tuberculous in origin until proven otherwise".

PLEURAL FLUID

The clinical types of pleural fluid collections are:
- *Pus*: Empyema or pyothorax
- *Serous fluid*: Hydrothorax
- *Blood*: Hemothorax
- *Chylous*: Chylothorax.

Empyema

Organisms: In the order of occurrence:
1. *Staphylococcus aureus*
2. *Haemophilus influenzae* type B
3. *Streptococcus pneumoniae*
4. *Klebsiellae*.

Clinical clues: Empyema is usually due to underlying pneumonia. Hence there will be features suggestive of pneumonia with features of fluid in the chest.

Clues for Staphylococcus Empyema

- Rapidly developing pleural fluid (pus) collection in less than 24 hours
- Development of pyopneumothorax
- Development of multiloculated empyema with or without loculated air pockets.

❒ Focal infections such as:
- Pustules
- Pyodermas
- Abscess
- Chronic suppurative otitis media
- Osteomyelitis of rib and spine
- Pyogenic arthritis in an infant
- Infected BCG wound
- Subdiaphragmatic infections such as hepatic or subphrenic abscess.

Though the most prevailing cause for empyema is *Staphylococcus aureus*, at times *Haemophilus influenzae*, and *Streptococcus pneumoniae* may be responsible for empyema.

Rapidly Developing Staphylococcal Empyema

❒ Vague opacification on the left lower lobe (Fig. 2.51).
❒ Repeat picture taken after 24 hours because of rapidly increasing respiratory distress shows developing empyema and more consolidating lower lobe pneumonia (Fig. 2.52).

Massive Empyema

Massive opacification of left side with shift of mediastinum (Fig. 2.53).

Clinical clues to rule out pleural effusion and consolidations are:
❒ Seriously ill, febrile, and toxic child
❒ Younger the age, especially infants
❒ Any extrapulmonary focal infections
❒ Possibility of consolidation of entire lung on one half is extremely rare.

Pyopneumothorax

❒ Air-fluid levels with massive opacification (Fig. 2.54)
❒ Multiseptated air pockets and air-fluid levels (Fig. 2.55).

Hydrothorax: Simple Pleural Effusion

Possible Causes

❒ Same organisms that produce empyema
❒ Viruses
❒ Tuberculosis
❒ Mycoplasma
❒ Renal—nephritis and nephrotic syndrome
❒ Abdominal tumors—neuroblastoma and lymphosarcoma
❒ Subphrenic or hepatic inflammations
❒ Chest wall or spine lesions

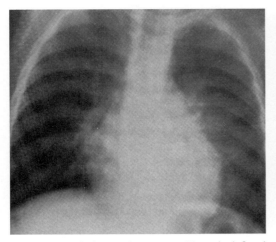

Fig. 2.51: Staphylococcal empyema. Vaguely defined infiltrate on the left, partially hidden by the heart.

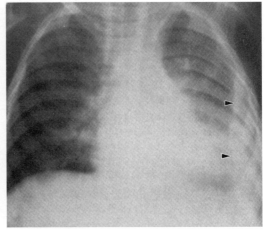

Fig. 2.52: Staphylococcal empyema. Within 24 hours there was rapidly developing empyema.

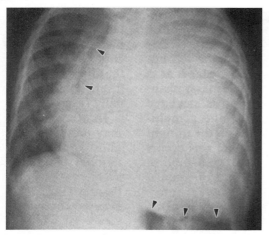

Fig. 2.53: Massive empyema. There is typical contralateral mediastinal shift and downward displacement of the left diaphragmatic leaflet and stomach.

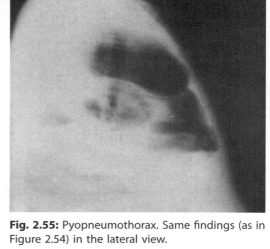

Fig. 2.55: Pyopneumothorax. Same findings (as in Figure 2.54) in the lateral view.

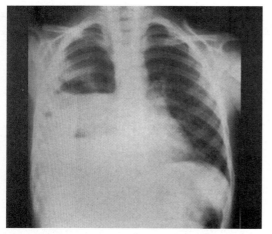

Fig. 2.54: Pyopneumothorax. Multiple septated fluid levels on the right characteristic of staphylococcal infection.

☐ Pancreatitis
☐ Congestive cardiac failure (CCF)
☐ Collagen vascular diseases.

Radiographic Types

Early or subtle pleural effusion: The earliest sign of minimal or subtle pleural effusion is that of blunting of costophrenic angle with wedge like menisci extending upward along the lateral border of chest wall. In the lateral view the same can be seen as curved or sloping menisci in the posterior costophrenic angle. Layering of fluid can also be seen at times on the retrosternal area.

Major or minor fissure opacification, other than a case of primary tuberculosis should invite attention to look for lateral layering as it often true to be due to pleural effusion.

Subtle or early or minimal effusion:
☐ *Fluid along the lateral chest wall (Fig. 2.56):* Right minor fissure opacification
☐ *Lateral view:* Thin layers of fluid in all the interlobar fissure. Layer of retrosternal fluid extension (Fig. 2.57).
☐ *Right lateral decubitus:* Shifts the fluid down to lateral chest wall and confirms the pleural fluid (Fig. 2.58).

Subtle effusion as vertical fissure opacification:
☐ When the fluid accumulates in the major fissure it can be seen as sloping vertical line either on the right or on the left
☐ Atelectasis of right upper lobe also present (Fig. 2.59).

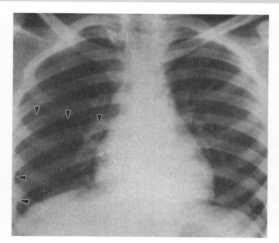

Fig. 2.56: Early, subtle pleural effusion. Thin layering of fluid in the right lateral chest wall and an indistinct extension into the minor fissure.

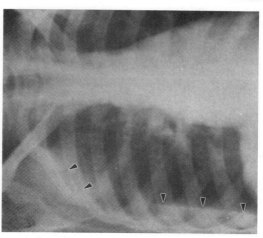

Fig. 2.58: Early, subtle pleural effusion. Right lateral decubitus view shows the real accumulated amount of fluid.

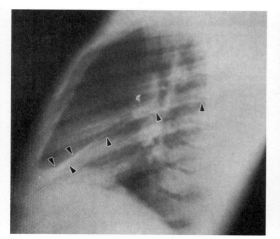

Fig. 2.57: Early, subtle pleural effusion. Lateral view showing all the interlobar fissures and a layer of fluid retrosternally.

Subtle interlobar fissure opacification:
- Parahilar peribronchial infiltrate (Fig. 2.60)
- Left lower lobe infiltrate
- Right hilum appears dense.

Lateral view shows triangular wedge-like opacification with posterior tapering running into minor fissure due to fluid accumulation (Fig. 2.61).

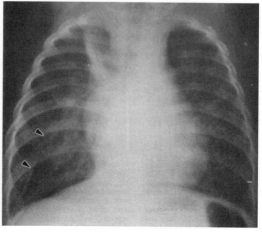

Fig. 2.59: Vertical fissure effusion. Accumulation of fluid in the lowermost portion of the major fissure gives an appearance of sloping vertical opacification. There is also an associated right upper lobe atelectasis.

Massive Pleural Effusion

Massive pleural effusion is usually not missed. They are characterized by:
- Massive opacification occupying not less than one-third of lung volume

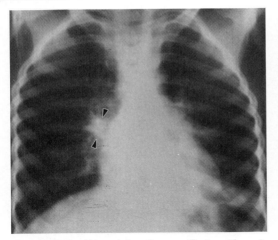

Fig. 2.60: Small interlobar fissure effusion. There is a viral left lower lobe infiltration with dense right hilum.

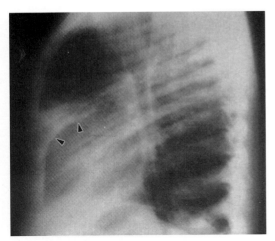

Fig. 2.61: Small interlobar fissure effusion. Triangular dense small anterior fissure effusion and posterior tapering as a wedge-like configuration as it runs along the minor fissure.

❑ Obliteration of costophrenic and cardiophrenic angles
❑ Shift of the mediastinum to the opposite side
❑ At times accompanied by:
  • Lateral layering extending into the apex
  • Encircling type of accumulation.

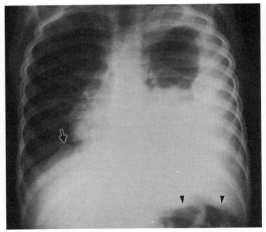

Fig. 2.62: Massive pleural effusion with large subpulmonic component. Massive left-sided effusion encircling the aerated lung with a large subpulmonic effusion depressing the stomach.

Subpulmonic Effusion Depressing the Diaphragmatic Leaflet

❑ Massive opacification occupying left half of the lung (Fig. 2.62)
❑ Lateral layering
❑ Encircling shadow extending into the apex and paraspinal gutter
❑ Shift of the mediastinum to the opposite side.

Mediastinal or Paraspinal Gutter Effusion

They often elude detection. Posteriorly they are seen as long, tapering, triangular or wedge-like paraspinal configuration.

Anteriorly they may look like mass-like or triangular shadow.

Mediastinal effusion: There is a triangular, right paramedian shadow with extension into minor fissure (Fig. 2.63).

Pleural Effusion with Pneumonia

There is a double opacified shadow with varying density (Fig. 2.64).

❑ Lower lobe consolidation seen as a slightly lesser in density

- Lateral vertical opacification with slightly increased density due to pleural fluid.

Large Pleural Effusion Mimicking Lobar Consolidation

Radiographic clues:

- The images may be round, oval, spindle-shaped or mass-like configuration
- Some may appear as irregular shadows
- Characteristic tapering ends when it involves the fissures

  Radiographic confirmation is by lateral decubitus view.

Pleural effusion mimicking lobar pneumonia:

- Curved elevation of opacification in the right lower half (Fig. 2.65)
- Lateral layering of fluid
- Minor fissure opacification.

Loculated Pleural Effusion

These groups of effusion may mimic consolidation and on lateral view the effusion could be confirmed.

- Large oval mass-like opacification on the right side sparing costophrenic and cardiophrenic angles (Fig. 2.66)
- Lateral view shows opacification in the axis of major fissure which confirms loculated effusion (Fig. 2.67)

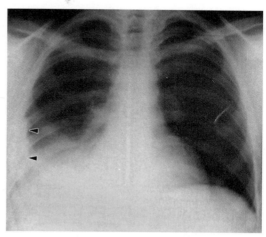

Fig. 2.64: Pneumonia with pleural effusion. There is an opacification in the right lower lobe due to consolidation and an additional layering in the lateral chest wall due to pleural effusion.

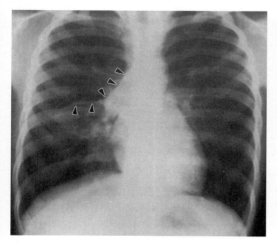

Fig. 2.63: Mediastinal effusion. Triangular configuration of fluid in the mediastinum and its extension into the minor fissure confirms the effusion.

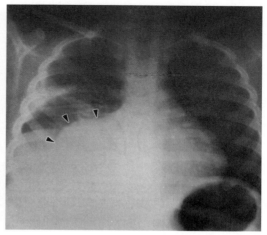

Fig. 2.65: Pleural effusion mimicking lobar pneumonia. The fluid along the right lateral chest wall and some fluid extending into the minor fissure confirm it to be pleural effusion.

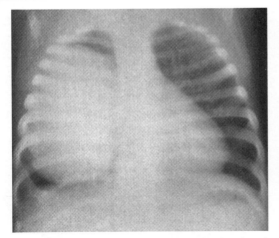

Fig. 2.66: Large loculated empyema. Large, loculated, perfectly oval, mass-like lesion of staphylococcal empyema.

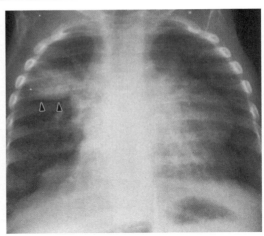

Fig. 2.68: Loculated pleural effusion. Posteroanterior view of the chest showing loculated effusion mimicking pneumonic consolidation.

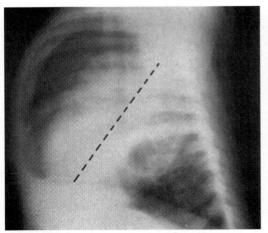

Fig. 2.67: Large loculated empyema. Lateral view showing mass-like lesion conforms to the axis of the major fissure.

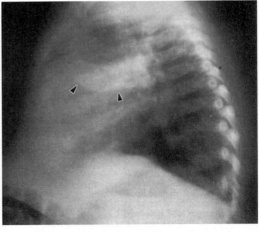

Fig. 2.69: Loculated pleural effusion. Lateral view showing pleural effusion loculated in the right minor fissure.

Loculated Effusion with Irregular Configuration

☐ Posteroanterior view shows opacification mimicking consolidation or segmental atelectasis (Fig. 2.68).
☐ Lateral view confirms the axis of opacification loculated in the minor fissure (Fig. 2.69).

Loculated Effusion in the Lateral Chest Wall

Oval-shaped effusion with adjacent consolidation possibly empyema in the resolving stage (Fig. 2.70).

Subpulmonic Effusions

They are difficult to detect unless otherwise one is aware of various radiographic clues

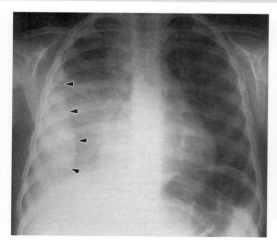 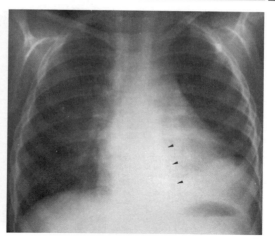

Fig. 2.70: Loculated effusion (lateral chest wall). Pneumonia evolving into empyema loculated laterally.

Fig. 2.71: Subpulmonic effusion. Apparently elevated left diaphragmatic leaflet with triangular strip of fluid in the paraspinal gutter with obliterated vascular markings through the left diaphragmatic leaflet.

consistent to the diagnosis. It may even mimic elevation of diaphragm. The possible radiographic clues are (Fig. 2.71):

❏ Unusual flatness of the apparently high diaphragmatic leaflet

❏ A sharp drop-off of the lateral edge of the diaphragmatic leaflet

❏ Obliteration of the adjacent portion of the cardiac silhouette

❏ Increased density of the posterior costophrenic recess

❏ Paraspinal collections of fluid, especially on the left

❏ Peculiar bumps and humps of the apparently high diaphragmatic leaflet.

❏ An increase in the space between the top of the apparently elevated diaphragmatic leaflet and stomach air bubble.

❏ Loss of visualization of the normal blood vessels of the lung through the upper most part of the apparent diaphragmatic leaflet.

HILAR AND PARATRACHEAL ADENOPATHY

The adenopathy in lungs are mostly inflammatory in origin. They can be unilateral or bilateral. The common causes of unilateral hilar or paratracheal adenopathy are:

❏ Viral LRTI

❏ Primary pulmonary tuberculosis.

At times adenopathy due to primary pulmonary tuberculosis may be associated with parenchymal infiltrate, atelectasis, and obstructive emphysema. A good rule of thumb to follow is that, "unilateral hilar or paratracheal adenopathy with or without associated changes in the lungs, should be considered tuberculous in origin until proven otherwise". The causes for bilateral adenopathy are commonly extrapulmonary such as sarcoidosis, histoplasmosis, histiocytosis, lymphoma, and leukemia. Parahilar peribronchial infiltrate with hilar adenopathy—typical of viral LRTI (Fig. 2.72).

❏ Unilateral paratracheal and hilar adenopathy of tuberculosis (Fig. 2.73)

❏ Unilateral hilar adenopathy with suspected atelectasis (Fig. 2.74)

• Lateral view confirms both atelectasis and paracarinal position of adenopathy (Fig. 2.75)

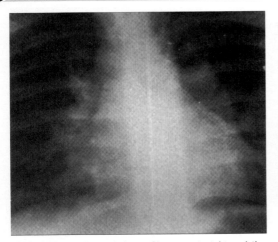

Fig. 2.72: Viral parahilar infiltrate mimicking hilar adenopathy. Parahilar peribronchial infiltrate with hilar adenopathy–typical of viral lower respiratory tract infection.

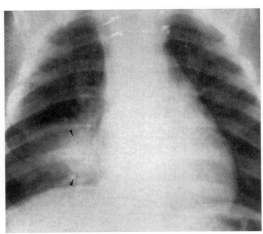

Fig. 2.74: Hilar adenopathy in tuberculosis hidden by atelectasis. Barely visible hilar adenopathy on the right hidden by right middle lobe atelectasis.

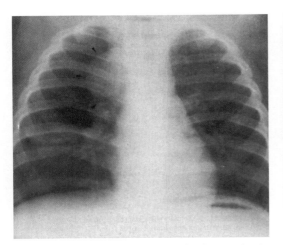

Fig. 2.73: Unilateral paratracheal adenopathy in tuberculosis. Extensive paratracheal adenopathy on the right.

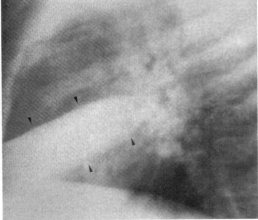

Fig. 2.75: Hilar adenopathy in tuberculosis hidden by atelectasis. Lateral view clearly shows the triangular dense atelectatic right middle lobe.

- ☐ Unilateral hilar adenopathy due to pulmonary tuberculosis (Fig. 2.76)
- ☐ Unilateral hilar adenopathy with obstructive emphysema on the left side (Fig. 2.77)
- ☐ Hilar adenopathy to differentiate from pneumonitis:

- Hilar adenopathy with central paracarinal position of opacification confirms the diagnosis (Figs. 2.78 and 2.79)
- The frontal hilar shadow on lateral view is located retrocarinal consistent with consolidation of superior segment of lower lobe (Figs. 2.80 and 2.81)

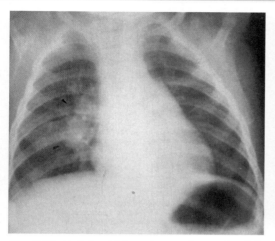

Fig. 2.76: Unilateral hilar adenopathy on the right due to tuberculosis.

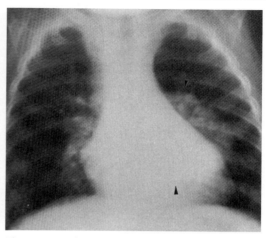

Fig. 2.78: Hilar adenopathy. There is a massive unilateral left hilar adenopathy in this patient with primary pulmonary tuberculosis.

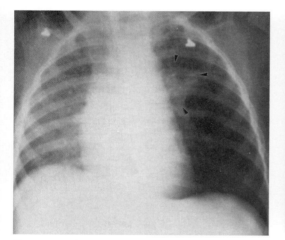

Fig. 2.77: Tuberculous adenopathy with obstructive emphysema. The expiratory film showing left-sided adenopathy and obstructive emphysema of the lung.

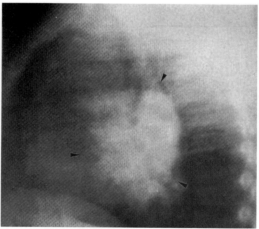

Fig. 2.79: Hilar adenopathy. Lateral view shows typical central, paracarinal location of hilar adenopathy.

ATELECTASIS

Atelectasis is a common X-ray finding and it can involve a small segment or one lobe or entire lung. The common causes are asthma, viral LRTI, primary tuberculosis or foreign bodies.

Certain radiographic rules to be followed in identifying atelectasis are:

❏ In obstructive emphysema, the large, hyperlucent lung will show ill-defined pulmonary vascularity.

❏ An obstructed emphysematous lung cannot compress upon the other lung to the point of total opacification.

❏ If a small totally opaque lung is seen it must be total atelectasis or agenesis of the lung

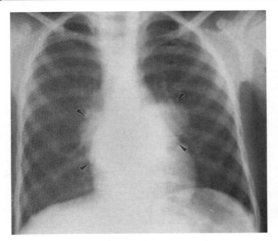

Fig. 2.80: Hilar adenopathy vs. Superior segment lower lobe pneumonia. This picture at first might suggest bilateral hilar adenopathy or a posterior mediastinal mass.

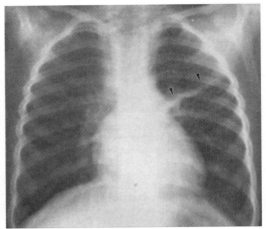

Fig. 2.82: Discoid or "plate-like" atelectasis. Segmental discoid atelectasis in the left upper lobe.

❏ The atelectatic segment or lobe in one view may be faintly visualized or nonvisualized and is clearly visualized in other view.

Segmental Atelectasis

They are often confused with pulmonary infiltrates or interlobar fissure effusion. Segmental atelectasis are often seen as "plate-like" or "disk-like". Segmental discoid atelectasis could be either single or multiple, vertical, horizontal or oblique.

❏ Segmental discoid atelectasis in the left upper lobe (Fig. 2.82)

❏ Vertical discoid atelectasis of left lower lobe (Fig. 2.83)

❏ Bilateral extensive multiple oblique discoid atelectasis (Fig. 2.84).

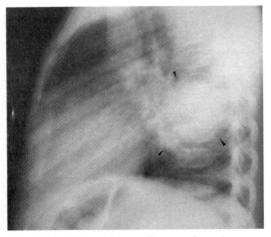

Fig. 2.81: Hilar adenopathy vs. Superior segment lower lobe pneumonia. In this lateral view the retrocarinal position of the lesion is in favor of bilateral superior segment lower lobe pneumonia.

❏ In a large, unobstructed emphysematous, hyperlucent lung the pulmonary vascularity is either normal or engorged

❏ The atelectatic lung will not change its size with phases of respiration

Total Lung Atelectasis

The features are:

❏ Total opacification of entire hemithorax

❏ Ipsilateral shift of mediastinum

❏ Heart hides into the atelectic lung. Total atelectasis of lung (Figs. 2.85 and 2.86):

• Marked loss of volume on the left side

• Marked shift of mediastinum to the left.

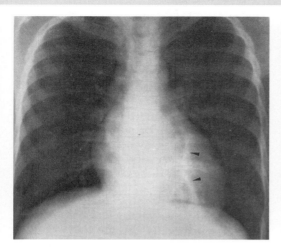

Fig. 2.83: Vertical discoid atelectasis. Segmental collapse occurring in vertical direction.

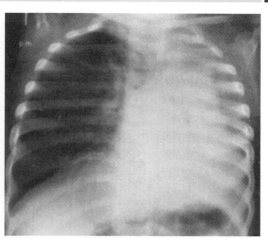

Fig. 2.85: Total lung atelectasis. Hyperlucent, retained vascularity on the right and loss of volume and mediastinal shift to the left due to mucus plugging in the left major bronchus.

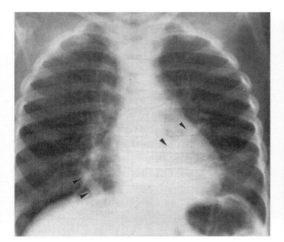

Fig. 2.84: Multiple discoid atelectasis. Bilateral multiple oblique densities representing multiple areas of segmental discoid atelectasis.

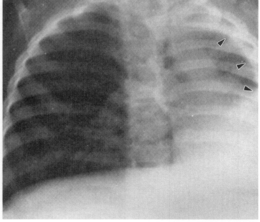

Fig. 2.86: Total lung atelectasis. Another patient with complete atelectasis of the left lung and pronounced compensatory emphysema of the right lung.

The pulmonary vascularity in the right lung is normal (compensatory emphysema).

Lobar Atelectasis of Right Side

Right Upper Lobe Atelectasis

The common classical features are (Fig. 2.87):

❑ Upper lobe is dense and triangular
❑ Minor fissure is elevated
❑ Slight mediastinal shift to the right—may or may not.

Lateral view shows characteristic wedged V-shaped configuration in between major and minor fissure (Fig. 2.88).

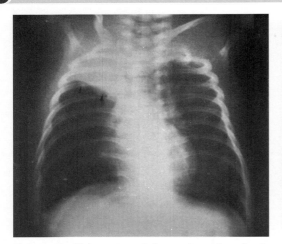

Fig. 2.87: Right upper lobe atelectasis—classic configuration.

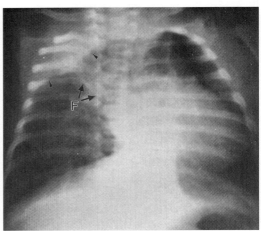

Fig. 2.89: Atypical right upper lobe atelectasis. Atelectatic right upper lobe compressed toward the apex of the right hemithorax and minor fissure is elevated.

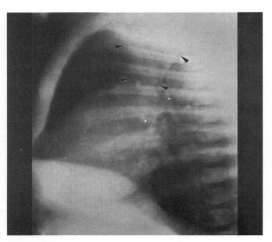

Fig. 2.88: Right upper lobe atelectasis. Lateral view of right upper lobe atelectasis demonstrating characteristic V–shaped configuration.

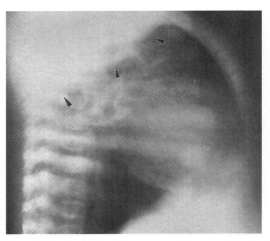

Fig. 2.90: Atypical right upper lobe atelectasis. Lateral view shows atypically collapsed right upper lobe in the apex of the heart.

Atypical Right Upper Lobe Collapse

The radiographic features are (Figs. 2.89 and 2.90):

- ❏ Compressed toward apex
- ❏ Minor fissure becomes indistinct but elevated
- ❏ Overaeration of middle and lower lobe.

Right Middle Lobe Collapse

The features are:

- ❏ Focal area of opacification along the lower right cardiac border
- ❏ Elevation of the right diaphragmatic leaflet
- ❏ Depression of right hilum

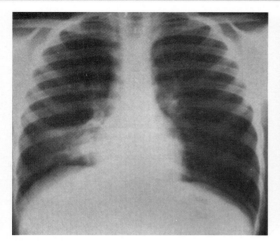

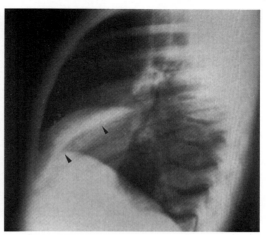

Fig. 2.91: Right middle lobe atelectasis. Classical findings are an area of increased density just to the right of the lower cardiac border, obliteration of the adjacent portion of the cardiac border, elevation of the diaphragmatic leaflet, and depression of the right hilum.

Fig. 2.92: Right middle lobe atelectasis. Lateral view shows the typical V-shaped configuration of the collapsed right middle lobe.

☐ On lateral view: typical inverted "V"-shaped opacification

☐ Slight shift of mediastinum to right (Figs. 2.91 and 2.92) presents with the all above features.

Right Upper and Middle Lobe Atelectasis

☐ Linear and diffuse opacification of medial portion of right lung
☐ Positive silhouette sign
☐ Smaller volume right hemithorax when compared to left
☐ Slight mediastinal shift to the right
☐ Mild elevation of right diaphragmatic leaflet
☐ Lateral view shows anterior displacement of major fissure with extended opacification in the region of upper and middle lobe with the lower most opacification is inverted "V" shape.

Right Lower Lobe Atelectasis

Dense triangular opacification starting retro-cardially at about the hilar level extending as curved outline beyond the right cardiac border merging with the right diaphragmatic leaflet.

☐ Slight elevation of right diaphragmatic leaflet
☐ Positive silhouette sign of right cardiac and right diaphragmatic border.
☐ Lateral view clearly visualized left dia-phragmatic leaflet and obliterated right leaflet with retrocardiac posterior most density.

Right Middle and Lower Lobe Atelectasis

Posteroanterior view: Dense triangular con-figuration starting at suprahilar level with straight sloping line toward the right costo-phrenic angle (Fig. 2.93).

Lateral view: Large area of increased density behind and over the heart (Fig. 2.94).

Left Lung Atelectasis

Left Upper Lobe Atelectasis

Since there is no minor fissure the lingula functions as part of left upper lobe and

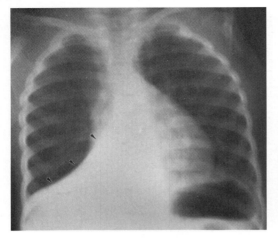

Fig. 2.93: Right lower lobe atelectasis. Dense triangular configuration of the collapsed right lower lobe with obliterated and elevated right diaphragmatic leaflet and a slight shift of the mediastinum to the right.

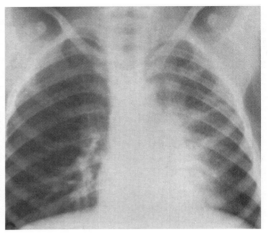

Fig. 2.95: Left upper lobe atelectasis. Left upper lobe and lingular atelectasis: shift of the mediastinum to the left, an obliteration of the entire left cardiac border. There is a diffuse central haziness of the left lung field.

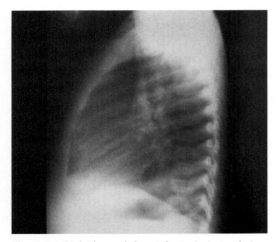

Fig. 2.94: Right lower lobe atelectasis. Lateral view shows a vague area of increased density.

atelectasis is seen as vague area of increased density and usually there will be associated secondary changes such as shift of the mediastinum and elevation of diaphragm.

Posteroanterior view: Left upper lobe and lingular atelectasis.

☐ Mediastinal shift to the left (Fig. 2.95)
☐ Positive silhouette sign by obliteration of left cardiac border
☐ Ill defined, vague, diffuse haziness over the left upper central lung field.

Lateral view: Collapsed lung with anterior displacement of major fissure (Fig. 2.96).

Left Lower Lobe Atelectasis

Classically it produces a triangular area of increased density, more or less confirmed to the area behind the left side of the heart.

There is a triangular area of opacification retrocardially and adjacent to the spine (Fig. 2.97).

As a general rule the pattern of atelectasis may vary from individual to individual depending upon the degree of atelectasis. Because of this, the familiarity with accessory signs such as displacement of hilum, shift of the mediastinum, and elevation of diaphragmatic leaflet will help us to arrive at a convincing conclusion.

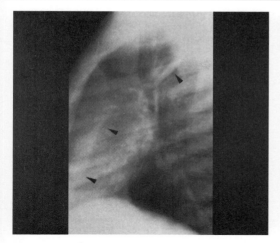

Fig. 2.96: Left upper lobe atelectasis. Lateral view shows the classic configuration of the collapsed upper lobe and lingula. The major fissure is displaced anteriorly.

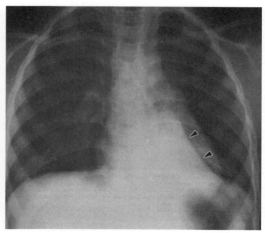

Fig. 2.97: Left lower lobe atelectasis. Classical triangular area of increased density behind the left side of the heart adjacent to the spine.

EMPHYSEMA

This may be either generalized or lobar. The cause for generalized emphysema is central obstructing lesions.

They are commonly:

- Tracheal foreign bodies
- Paratracheal masses
- Vascular rings
- Viral or thermal induced injury with air trapping
- Asthmatic bronchospasm
- Cystic fibrosis
- Rarely alpha-1 antitrypsin deficiency.

Radiographic clues:

- Overdistended, overaerated lungs
- Abnormal tracheal deviation
- Right-sided aortic arch with the possibility of aortic vascular ring
- Mediastinal mass.

Endotracheal Opaque Foreign Bodies

Lateral view (Fig. 2.98):

- Overdistended chest

- Typical bell-shaped configuration. PA view (Fig. 2.99)
- Overaerated hyperlucent lungs
- Extremely depressed diaphragm with a sloping sweep.

Lobar Emphysema

- Usually congenital since birth
- May become symptomatic by adulthood
- May present as respiratory distress syndrome after or at the time of simple respiratory infection
- Commonly seen in the left upper lobe
- Can also occur in right upper lobe and middle lobe
- Lower lobe involvement is very rare
- May mimic congenital cystic adenomatoid malformation.

Congenital Left Upper Lobe Emphysema

- Hyperlucent left upper lobe (Fig. 2.100)
- Small triangular collapsed left lower lobe
- Mediastinal shift to the right.

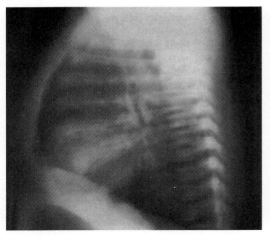

Fig. 2.98: Obstructive emphysema. Lateral view of emphysematous lung with increased antero-posterior diameter assuming bell shape and flat diaphragmatic leaflets.

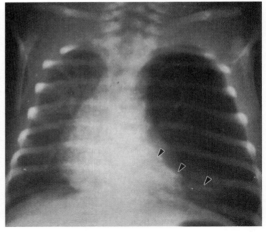

Fig. 2.100: Congenital lobar emphysema. Hyper-lucent left upper lobe and small triangularly collapsed lower lobe.

❒ Fluid free
❒ Single or multiple
❒ Some may rapidly change in size to rupture and produce pneumothoraces
❒ Some may remain static for extended periods of time
❒ The common cause is staphylococcal pneumonia.
   Rarely may be due to viral LRTI, tuberculosis, hydrocarbon pneumonia, closed or blunt chest trauma.
❒ Large pneumatocele with adjacent small pneumatocele in the right lower lobe (Fig. 2.101).
❒ 7 days later numerous and larger size pneumatoceles are found since not responding to antibiotic (Fig. 2.102).

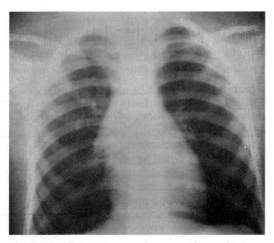

Fig. 2.99: Obstructive emphysema. Thermal injury-induced bronchiolitis due to smoke inhalation behaving as obstruction leading to emphysematous overaeration.

PNEUMATOCELES AND PULMONARY ABSCESS

Pneumatocele

❒ Thin-walled air-filled cyst
❒ Variable in size

Pulmonary Abscess

They are commonly due to complications of pneumonias or chronic bronchial obstruction with suppuration. The features are:
❒ Thick-walled lesions
❒ Regular or irregular in outline
❒ Round or oval in shape

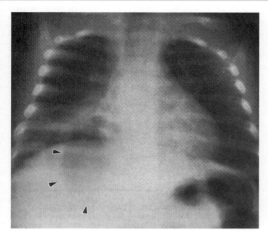

Fig. 2.101: Staphylococcal pneumonia with pneumatocele. Medial large pneumatocele with a small superior pneumatocele.

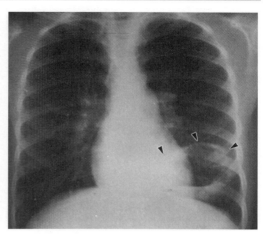

Fig. 2.103: Pulmonary abscess. Rounded pus-filled abscess in the left lung with air fluid level in the bottom of the abscess.

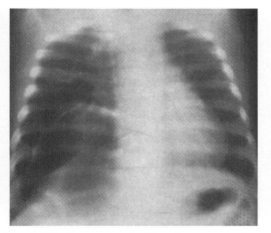

Fig. 2.102: Pneumatocele. The picture was taken 7 days after the first picture (Fig. 2.101) evolving into a larger pneumatocele and many other small pneumatocele adjacent to it. There is a mild shift of the mediastinum to the left.

❏ Air fluid levels are significant
❏ PA—thick walled, irregular appearing cavity in the left lower lobe (Fig. 2.103)
❏ Air fluid level is seen (Fig. 2.104).

Air Trappings in the Chest

The causes of air trappings in the chest are:

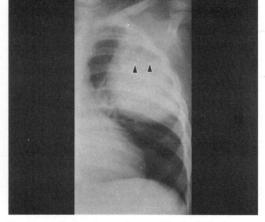

Fig. 2.104: Pulmonary abscess. Thick-walled irregular appearing abscess in the left lower lobe with air-fluid level in the bottom of the abscess.

❏ Closed or penetrating chest trauma
❏ Asthma
❏ Pulmonary infections
❏ Obstructing lesions of the airway such as:
  • Foreign bodies
  • Vascular rings
  • Mediastinal cysts
  • Masses.

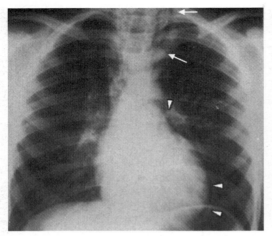

Fig. 2.105: Pneumomediastinum. Pneumomediastinal air surrounding the small triangular thymus, extending in linear sheaths into the neck and superior mediastinum and extending along the lower left cardiac edge.

Fig. 2.106: Pneumomediastinum. Pneumomediastinal air outlining the thymus on the left and clearly and continuously visible diaphragm producing the "continuous diaphragmatic sign".

Pneumomediastinum

- Central in location
- Occupies various shapes and sizes
- Usually outlines the mediastinal structures such as thymus, aorta, and pulmonary artery
- Free air can extend upward to outline the great vessels and soft tissues of the superior mediastinum and neck
- At times it may outline the heart.
- May get collected subpleurally along the diaphragm producing "continuous diaphragm sign".
- Air outlining the mediastinal structures such as thymus and heart (Fig. 2.105).
- Entire width of diaphragm is seen from side to side lifting the heart slightly above (Fig. 2.106).

Pneumothorax

Radiographic clues:
- Increased size and lucency of the involved hemithorax

- Contralateral shift of the mediastinum
- Increased sharpness of the ipsilateral mediastinal edge
- Lateral or decubitus view in suspected doubtful cases show air occupying the top most column
- Unaltered volume and lucency of the affected chest on expiration
- Absent vascular markings on the involved side
- Subtle or small pneumothorax on careful scrutinization over its apex or costophrenic angle delineates the small air pockets.
  - In the apex it is seen as a slender, radiolucent apical cap.
  - In the costophrenic angle typical, laterally pointing v-shaped air fluid level is seen.

Pneumopericardium

Usually following a history of penetrating type of chest wall injury the pneumopericardium may occur. It is an ectopic gas in

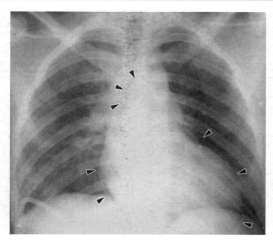

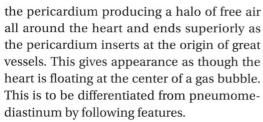

Fig. 2.107: Traumatic pneumoperitoneum. A halo of free air around the heart also extending along the aorta.

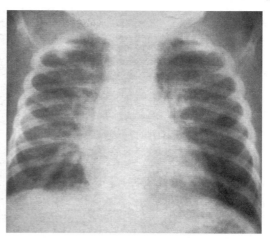

Fig. 2.108: Pneumonitis. Parahilar peribronchial infiltrate with normal heart due to viral pneumonitis.

the pericardium producing a halo of free air all around the heart and ends superiorly as the pericardium inserts at the origin of great vessels. This gives appearance as though the heart is floating at the center of a gas bubble. This is to be differentiated from pneumomediastinum by following features.

❑ Pneumopericardium does not outline the thymus with gas.

❑ Pneumopericardium does not extend superiorly beyond the origin of the great vessels.

❑ A halo of free air around the heart (Fig. 2.107)

❑ Air extending along the aorta.

PULMONARY CONGESTION AND PULMONARY EDEMA

Pulmonary congestion and edema can rise from a number of cardiac and noncardiac causes. In arriving at a radiographic diagnosis of pulmonary edema one must keep in mind certain basic anatomical and hemodynamic events which help pediatrician to have a precise approach.

The most important point in differentiation between viral LRTI, parahilar pneumonitic infiltrate with that of pulmonary edema is cardiomegaly.

Pneumonia versus Pulmonary Congestion

❑ Parahilar peribronchial infiltrate of viral LRTI without cardiomegaly (Fig. 2.108)

❑ Cardiomegaly with pulmonary congestion (Fig. 2.109).

PULMONARY CONGESTION

They are of two types:
1. Active congestion
2. Passive congestion.

Active congestion in an L—R shunt usually of congenital heart disease results in more blood flow into the lungs and, hence, the arteries enlarge and tortuous and visualized up to the periphery.

On the other hand passive congestion is mainly due to left heart failure, and so flow into the lungs are not significant but the increased pulmonary venous pressure leads to distension of pulmonary veins

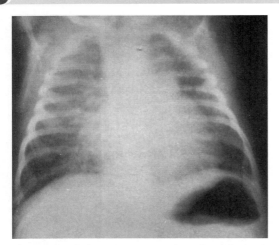

Fig. 2.109: Pulmonary congestion. Parahilar pulmonary congestion with enlarged heart due to heart disease.

and capillaries, followed by oozing out of fluid into the perivascular interstitium (fuzzy appearance of vessels and Kerley's A and B line) and finally leading to alveolar accumulation of fluid. This alveolar fluid collection, when it occupies the parahilar region, produces typical "butterfly" configuration with clear periphery or may produce pulmonary consolidation either nodular or lobar type. The causes for such type of passive congestion are:

- Obstructing lesions in aortic stenosis and coarctation of aorta
- Myocardial dysfunction such as myocarditis, endocardial fibroelastosis, and rheumatic fever
- Acute glomerulonephritis (AGN)
- Iatrogenic fluid over load
- Smoke or hot air inhalation
- Noxious fume inhalation
- Near drowning
- Rheumatic pneumonia
- Collagen vascular disease
- Massive aspiration
- Fat embolism

- Allergic pneumonitis
- Neurogenic pulmonary edema secondary to increased intracranial pressure
- Shock lung syndrome
- Poisoning by heroin, methadone, librium, carbon monoxide, and parathion.

STAGES OF PULMONARY EDEMA

Interstitial Stage

First development of interstitial stage radiographically is streaky or reticular white lines in the chest, followed by increasing generalized opacity or haziness of the lungs and commonly are referred to as Kerley "A" and "B" lines. The "B" lines are the small, transverse lines located in the costophrenic sulci and the "A" lines are the longer lines, generally running outward from the hilar regions.

Alveolar Stage

After saturation of interstitium with the fluid, it oozes out into the alveolar space producing consolidation like picture of nodular or diffuse haziness. When it accumulates in parahilar region with the clear periphery it gives "butterfly" appearance.

In many of the cases edema results from the damaging of the capillaries with the resultant increased permeability and extravasations of fluid into the interstitial and alveolar spaces. In increased intracranial pressure due to associated bradycardia and low cardiac output, there is elevated pulmonary venous and arterial pressure. This increased hydrostatic pressure leads to capillary extravasation of fluid into the surrounding lung.

In near drowning it is mainly direct aspiration of liquid into the lung parenchyma that produces edema.

In smoke and noxious fume inhalation, bronchiolar epithelial injury initially causes air trapping and later replaced by nonspecific infiltrates as a result of microatelectasis secondary to pulmonary microembolization. Necrotizing bronchiolitis is one another mechanism which leads to rapid development of pulmonary edema with the resultant fatality.

In rheumatic pneumonia, the streptococcal toxin by damaging and increasing the pulmonary capillary permeability, the pulmonary edema develops.

In fat embolism, it is trapping of the fat droplets in the microcirculation of pulmonary vessels those results in pulmonary edema.

In shock lung due to profound hypoxia and hypotension neurogenic pulmonary edema occurs.

Pulmonary Edema–Interstitial Stage

☐ A case of AGN with white streaky lines radiating from the hilum—Kerley "A" lines (Fig. 2.110).

☐ A case of cardiac failure due to aortic stenosis with extensive reticular pattern (Fig. 2.111).

☐ A case of AGN, with extensive reticulation in the lung with Kerley "B" lines in the costophrenic angle (Fig. 2.112).

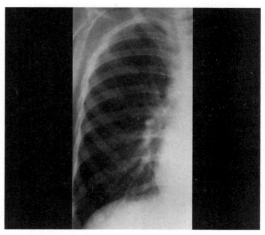

Fig. 2.110: Pulmonary edema—interstitial stage. Radiating streaky white lines from hilum—Kerley "A" lines in a patient with acute glomerulonephritis.

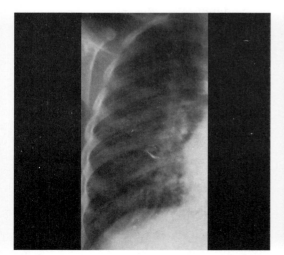

Fig. 2.111: Pulmonary edema—interstitial stage. Extensive reticular pattern of pulmonary interstitial edema in a patient with cardiac failure.

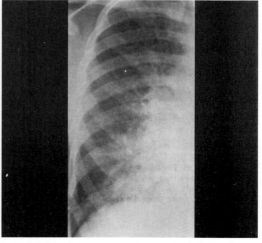

Fig. 2.112: Pulmonary edema—interstitial stage. More extensive pronounced reticulation due to severe interstitial edema with Kerley "B" lines.

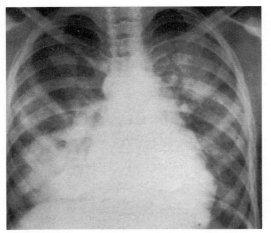

Fig. 2.113: Pulmonary edema—alveolar stage. Bilateral extensive patchy areas of confluent pulmonary alveolar edema.

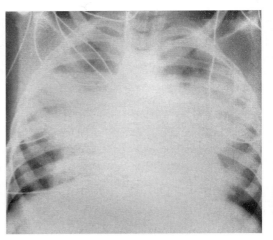

Fig. 2.114: Pulmonary alveolar edema. The pulmonary alveolar edema in Parahilar and midlung field and apical sparing gives an appearance of typical "butterfly" configuration.

Pulmonary Edema–Alveolar Stage

❏ Bilateral extensive, atypical patchy confluent pulmonary edema (Fig. 2.113)
❏ Prominent parahilar "butterfly" type pulmonary edema sparing the apices and costophrenic and cardiophrenic angles (Fig. 2.114).

ASTHMATIC CHEST

Diagnosing asthma is not a challenging one and does not always warrant X-ray chest. It is the complication and differentiating asthma mimicking situations is more important than diagnosing classical clinical asthma.

The underlying pathogenetic mechanisms are bronchospasm, mucosal edema, and increased viscid mucosal secretions with impending mucosal plugging.

The spectrums of radiographic images are:
❏ Typical baseline asthmatic chest
❏ Atelectasis mimicking pneumonia in asthma
❏ Pneumomediastinum
❏ Pneumothorax
❏ Obstructive emphysema
❏ Compensatory emphysema

❏ Prominent pulmonary artery
❏ Transient peripleural focal atelectasis.

Typical Baseline Asthmatic Chest

The presentation are widespread overaeration, parahilar peribronchial prominence, and bronchial cuffing with or without hilar adenopathy. The picture may almost mimic that of viral LRTI and the only clue is recurrence of episodes and occurrence at times may be without fever.
❏ Overaeration of lung (Fig. 2.115)
❏ Prominent parahilar peribronchial infiltration
❏ Bronchial cuffing
❏ Hilar adenopathy.

Lateral view (Fig. 2.116):
❏ Overdistended chest
❏ Increased retrosternal depth with the heart.

Atelectasis Mimicking Pneumonia in Asthma

Wheezing episodes at time may be associated with LRTI, but more often it is viral than

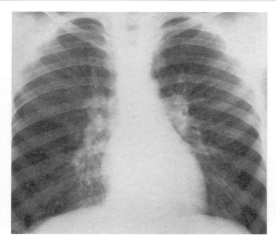

Fig. 2.115: Typical baseline asthmatic chest. Moderately overaerated lung with parahilar peribronchial infiltrate, bronchial cuffing and hilar adenopathy.

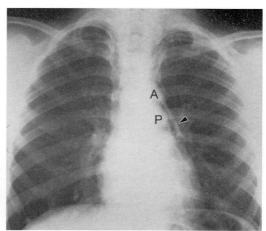

Fig. 2.117: Asthmatic pneumomediastinum. Pneumomediastinal air outlining the aorta (A), pulmonary artery (P) and a slender left thymic lobe (arrowhead).

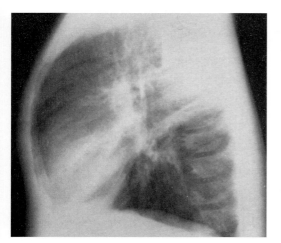

Fig. 2.116: Typical baseline asthmatic chest. Overdistended chest and pushed away heart from the sternum.

bacterial. Certain significant clinical observations are:

❏ Viral infections are more common than bacterial

❏ Increase in wheezing is more common in viral than bacterial

❏ Bacterial infections are usually parenchymal and viral infections are peribronchial.

Though the possibility for bacterial infections is there in an asthmatic child, it is the viral, inflammatory mucus plugging with transient segmental atelectasis is more common than that of bacterial in origin. For the same reason obstructive and compensatory emphysemas are also common in asthmatic child.

Pneumomediastinum Complicating Asthma

❏ Pneumomediastinal air outlining the aorta and pulmonary artery (Fig. 2.117)

❏ *Lateral view*: Thymus gland is surrounded by pneumomediastinal air (Fig. 2.118).

Obstructive Emphysema

Inspiratory film (Fig. 2.119):

❏ Hyperaerated lung

❏ Overdistension of lung by virtue of low placed diaphragm.

Expiratory film (Fig. 2.120):

❏ Partial emptying of lung

❏ Shift of mediastinum to the left

❏ Unaltered right lung.

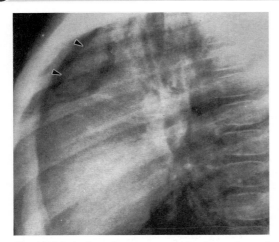

Fig. 2.118: Asthmatic pneumomediastinum. Lateral view in an asthmatic patient showing a small thymus surrounded by pneumomediastinal air.

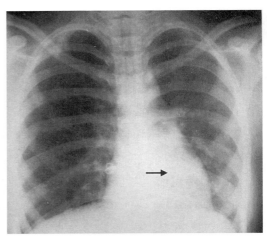

Fig. 2.120: Mucus plug causing unsuspected obstructive emphysema. Expiratory film showing shift of the mediastinum to the left with the possibility of mucus plug obstruction.

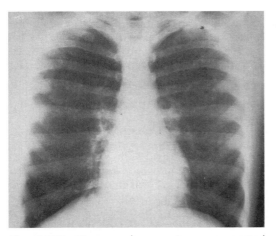

Fig. 2.119: Mucous plug causing unsuspected obstructive emphysema. Inspiratory film showing bilateral overaeration tempting to interpret as normal.

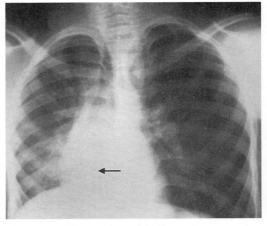

Fig. 2.121: Mucus plug with distracting contralateral compensatory emphysema. Inspiratory film showing mediastinal shift to the right and compensatory overaeration of left lung.

Hence, there is an obstructive emphysema on the right side.

Compensatory Emphysema

Inspiratory film (Fig. 2.121):
□ Marked mediastinal shift to the right
□ Overaeration of left lung.

Expiratory film (Fig. 2.122):
□ Left lung is emptied
□ Heart replaced partially to the left
□ Unaltered right lung.

Hence, there is possibility of mucus plug obstructing on the right with the compensatory emphysema on the left.

Prominent Pulmonary Artery

Prominent pulmonary artery possibly due to acute pulmonary hypertension (Fig. 2.123).

Elongated Small Heart

❏   Bilateral overaeration of lung (Fig. 2.124)
❏   Long thin cardiac silhouette.

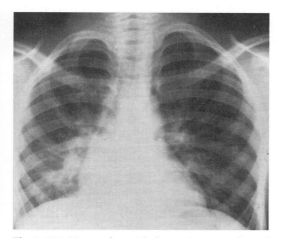

Fig. 2.122: Mucus plug with distracting contralateral compensatory emphysema. Expiratory film shows emptied lung on the left and maintaining the same position on the right possibly due to mucus plug on the right.

█ COMMON IN STATUS ASTHMATICUS

Foreign Bodies in the Lower Airway

Small infants by virtue of their habit of taking anything on their way into the mouth are highly prone for foreign body aspiration into the airway. Whenever a child who is just previously normal in all aspect suddenly develops violent coughing, gagging and vomiting, and varying degrees of respiratory distress and at times even cyanosis, one must strongly suspect foreign body aspiration.

Sometimes all the clinical symptoms may quickly resolve with or without vomiting the foreign body even then one must not be distracted away from evaluation, because undetected foreign body may go in for recurrent pneumonias or wheezing suggestive of asthma. Of course, sudden onset of wheezing in a previously unknown history should be considered due to foreign body or another obstructing lesion such as vascular ring until proven otherwise.

The most important thing in foreign bodies' evaluation is, once you start suspecting, you must proceed working up which

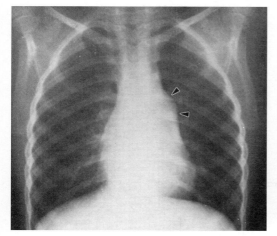

Fig. 2.123: Prominent pulmonary artery in asthma.

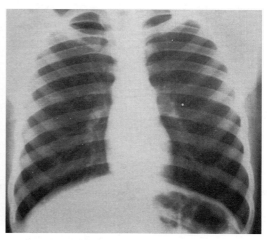

Fig. 2.124: Elongated small heart in asthma.

must be immediate and thorough until you prove or disprove it.

The radiographic features may vary from normal lung to one that of pneumomediastinum and pneumothorax. One another problem that we encounter is radiolucent foreign body which evades evaluation. So it is the indirect evidence which may mimic lot of other conditions like pneumonia, atelectasis, and asthma and a skillful pediatrician must be alert enough to correlate the clinical events and radiography. The sincere follow up is equally important in clinching the diagnosis.

The spectrum of radiographic pictures could be:

- Opaque foreign body anywhere in the respiratory tract
- Normal lung
- Obstructive emphysema
- Compensatory emphysema
- Atelectasis
- Air trapping such as pneumothorax and pneumomediastinum
- Pneumonitic patches (acute and recurrent)
- Bronchiectasis (in neglected cases).

The most common radiographic picture encountered is obstructive emphysema. Most of the time, physiologic dilatation of bronchus during inspiration and ball valve effect of foreign bodies allows the air to be trapped in the distal lung. With the ongoing respiratory cycle there is eventual accumulation of air and the affected side lung appears larger and hyperlucent. Ultimately pulmonary blood flow is also compromised.

Inspiratory film (Fig. 2.125):

- Obstructive emphysema due to foreign body in the left mainstem bronchus
- Large hyperlucent right lung
- Oligemia of the right lung
- Mediastinal shift to the left
- Downward displacement of left diaphragmatic leaflet.

Expiratory film (Fig. 2.126):

- All the above features are accentuated
- Significant shift of the mediastinum to the left
- Normal left lung has partially emptied the air and, hence, significantly deflated.

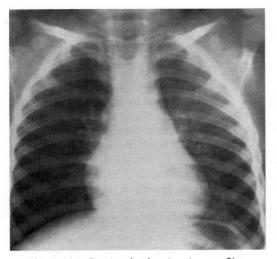

Fig. 2.125: Foreign body—inspiratory film.

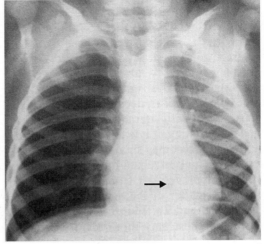

Fig. 2.126: Foreign body—expiratory film.

Foreign Body Mimicking Pneumonia

- Infiltrate in the left lower lobe (Fig. 2.127)
- Compensatory emphysema of left upper lobe.

Next day film (as the symptoms worsened):
- Features of obstructive emphysema (Fig. 2.128)
- Underlying peanut fragments were removed.

Right Lower Lobe Atelectasis (Fig. 2.129)

Compensatory emphysema of right upper lobe and entire left lung

Expiratory film (Fig. 2.130):
- Partial to near emptying of normal right upper lobe and entire left lung
- No air trapping anywhere
- Persistence of atelectasis of right lower lobe (A tack was identified and removed).

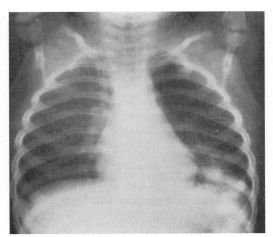

Fig. 2.127: Foreign body disguised as pneumonia.

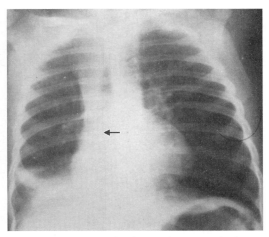

Fig. 2.129: Foreign body producing right lower lobe atelectasis.

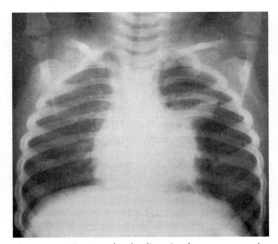

Fig. 2.128: Foreign body disguised as pneumonia.

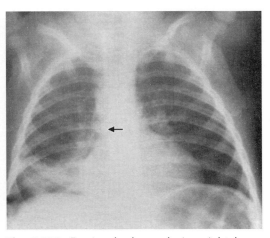

Fig. 2.130: Foreign body producing right lower lobe atelectasis.

Foreign Body with Pneumomediastinum

❑ Extensive free air in the mediastinum, soft tissues of the neck and chest (Fig. 2.131)
❑ Right lung is slightly emphysematous
❑ Air trapping is to be suspected because of foreign body in the right main bronchus.

MISCELLANEOUS CHEST PROBLEMS

Aspiration Problems

By virtue of ignorance and immaturity during the period of infancy, the aspiration of various substances may occur accidentally. The aspirations may be substance-related or defect-related events.

Substances: The common substance which may induce chemical pneumonitis even with few drops are hydrocarbons which include furniture polish, kerosene, gasoline, etc. The other substances aspirated may be milk, food, and for that matter any liquid that is taken by the child.

Defects: The anatomical and physiological defects such as swallowing mechanism defect, tracheoesophageal fistulae, seizures, gastroesophageal reflux with or without underlying hiatus hernia.

Radiographic Features

This could be pneumonia which can be focal or widespread and the findings depend on the volume of the fluid aspirated and the position of the patient at the time of aspiration. Certain radiographic features which are often seen are:

❑ In small infants, who are fed in lying posture are prone for right upper lobe involvement.
❑ Aspiration in the upright position leads to medially positioned lower lobe infiltrates which may mimic hydrocarbon aspiration.
❑ Massive aspiration may mimic those of pulmonary edema or extensive bacterial pneumonia.
❑ Chronic and recurrent aspiration problems may lead on to fibrosis, bronchitis and even bronchiectasis.
❑ Chronic lipid aspiration often leads to very dense, hazy lungs.
❑ In hydrocarbon aspiration, the pulmonary changes are absent for the first 6–12 hours. After that local effects of lipid dissolution and cell membrane destruction occur rapidly and hyperemia, edema, bronchial and bronchiolar necrosis, peribronchial edema, small vessel thrombosis, and necrotizing bronchopneumonia soon develop. The hydrocarbon being lipid solvent, destroys surfactant and leads to microatelectasis of the alveoli.

Radiographically infiltrates develop in the lung bases medially and may range from minimal fluffy infiltrates to dense streaky nodular or confluent infiltrates involving a good portion of the lungs bilaterally.

In few cases a severe form of injury may develop into focal emphysema, pleural effusion, and pneumatocele.

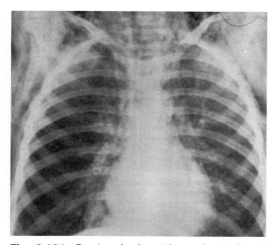

Fig. 2.131: Foreign body with mediastinal and interstitial air.

Right Upper Lobe Atelectasis (Fig. 2.132)

❑ Collapsed upper lobe is dense and triangular
❑ Minor fissure is elevated
❑ Minimal mediastinal shift to the right.

This can occur in infants with aspiration in lying posture.

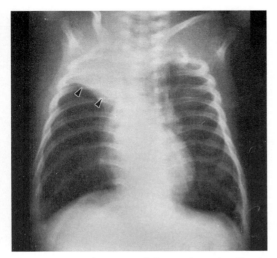

Fig. 2.132: Right upper lobe atelectasis. Classic configuration of triangularly collapsed upper lobe and elevated minor fissure collapse.

Lateral view (Fig. 2.133): V-shaped configuration of the collapsed right upper lobe. The collapsed lobe is delineated anteriorly by minor fissure and posteriorly by major fissure.

Hydrocarbon pneumonitis in upright position (Red furniture polish):

❑ 2 hours after ingestion (Fig. 2.134): Radiographically normal lung.
❑ By 12 hours (Fig. 2.135): Extensive bilateral typical infiltrates in the lung bases medially.

Chronic Lipoid Aspiration

Dense, diffuse, hazy infiltrates in both lungs secondary to lipid aspiration (Fig. 2.136).

Overaerated Lung with Microcardia

Hyperinflated lung with stretched out heart may occur in so many clinical conditions.

The most common being dehydration with acidosis. Here, because of hyperventilation in an acidotic child in an attempt to blow off carbon dioxide, the lungs are overaerated, which depresses the diaphragmatic leaflet and stretches out the heart and the lungs are under vascularized.

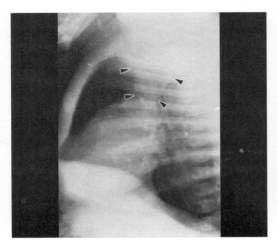

Fig. 2.133: Right upper lobe atelectasis. Lateral view of classic configuration as V-shaped.

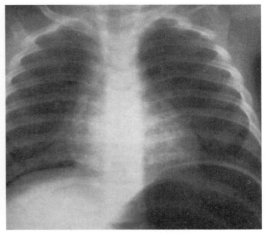

Fig. 2.134: Hydrocarbon pneumonia. At the end of 2 hours of aspiration of furniture polish.

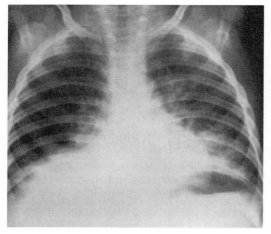

Fig. 2.135: Hydrocarbon pneumonia. After 12 hours, typical bilateral extensive basal medial infiltrate.

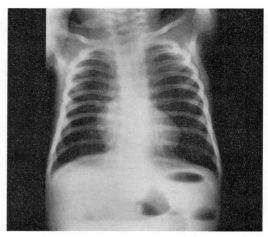

Fig. 2.137: Hyperlucent overaerated lung in a child with diarrheal dehydration.

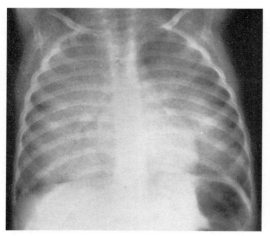

Fig. 2.136: Lipoid aspiration pneumonia. Bilateral dense hazy infiltrate.

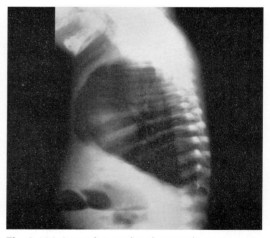

Fig. 2.138: Lateral view also showing hyperaeration without expansion of anteroposterior diameter unlike in a bronchiolitis.

This occurs in dehydration following acute gastroenteritis.

Overaeration in a dehydrated child (Fig. 2.137):
- ❑ Lungs are overdistended
- ❑ Lungs are overaerated and so hyperlucent
- ❑ Diminished vascularity
- ❑ Depressed diaphragmatic leaflet

- ❑ Slightly elongated heart (microcardia). Lateral view showing emphysematous lungs.

Overdistended lung with microcardia can also occur in acute large blood volume loss (Fig. 2.138). Some other causes of microcardia are Addison's disease, anorexia nervosa, long thin normal asthenic individual, and long-standing debilitating diseases such as malignancy, malnutrition, severe burns, and chronic infections.

Allergic Pneumonitis

The lung involvement due to allergy can occur in two important situations. It may be either toxic substance inhalation or cytotoxic drug ingestion (especially following cancer therapy). The resultant infiltrates may be focal or generalized depending upon the amount of the substances either inhaled or ingested. They are usually waxing and waning in nature especially with steroid therapy.

Bilateral extensive hazy infiltrate following leukemic therapy (Fig. 2.139). 24 hours after administration of steroids the lungs became clear.

Lung and Hemoptysis

Though not common, hemoptysis may occur in:
- ❑ Hemangiomas of airway
- ❑ Foreign bodies in the airway
- ❑ Bronchial adenomas
- ❑ Intrathoracic gastroenteric cysts

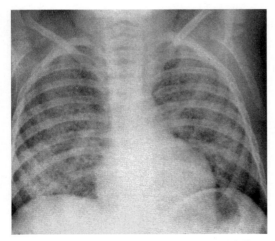

Fig. 2.139: Bilateral extensive hazy infiltrate following leukemic therapy with cytotoxic drugs.

- ❑ Chronic pulmonary infections
- ❑ Pulmonary hemosiderosis.

Radiographic presentations could be anything from miliary like nodules, discrete cystic masses, and fluffy bilateral infiltrates to nonspecific consolidative lesions.

Pulmonary hemosiderosis: Radiological findings include fluffy, asymmetric infiltrate resembling widespread pneumonias or even pulmonary edema and rarely diffuse miliary infiltrate.

Delayed Diaphragmatic Hernia

Classically the diaphragmatic hernia occurs as an acute newborn emergency with respiratory distress. Very rarely in older children one of the causes of acute respiratory distress could be due to delayed herniation of stomach or intestinal contents either through an existing congenital diaphragmatic defect or through an acquired defect following blunt abdominal trauma either on an acute or delayed basis.

Very often it is misinterpreted as large pneumothorax or cystic mass, unless one is concentrating on the continuity of bowel shadows into the thorax or confirming by barium meal series.
- ❑ Large hyperlucent mass in the left hemithorax
- ❑ Mediastinal shift to the right (Fig. 2.140)
- ❑ Absence of stomach air bubble.
- ❑ Continuation of bowel gas shadow into the involved thorax.

Chest Masses

The most important things to be kept in mind to evaluate radiologically intrathoracic mass or cysts are:
- ❑ Clinically chest pain, respiratory distress, wheezing or asthma-like symptoms
- ❑ Possible rapid expansion with accentuation of clinical symptoms
- ❑ Nonresponse to conventional management

❏ The size of the lesion is relatively larger than commonly seen.

Some of the common masses are mediastinal lymphomas, thymus gland infiltrated with leukemic cells, and pulmonary cysts.

❏ Large mediastinal mass presenting as superior mediastinal widening—clinically presenting as wheezing. Biopsy-proven lymphoma (Fig. 2.141)

❏ Clinically asthma like (Fig. 2.142):
  • Large mass in the left hemithorax with calcification
  • Biopsy proven teratoma
❏ Clinically respiratory distress (Fig. 2.143):
  • Large mass on the right side with air pockets
  • Biopsy-proven infected bronchogenic cyst.

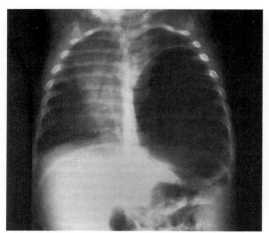

Fig. 2.140: Delayed presentation of a diaphragmatic hernia in an older child mimicking cyst-like lesion.

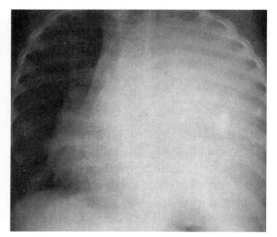

Fig. 2.142: Teratoma. Note a large mass with calcification in the left chest who was screened for asthma-like symptoms.

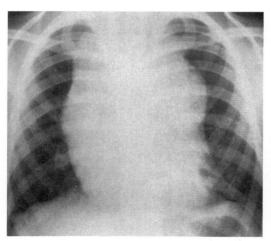

Fig. 2.141: Rapidly expanding mass. This large mass which was interpreted as pneumonia was found to be a case of rapidly expanding mass of lymphoma.

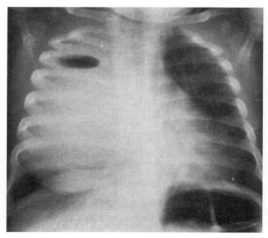

Fig. 2.143: Large infected bronchogenic cyst. Bronchogenic cyst compressing the trachea and right bronchus.

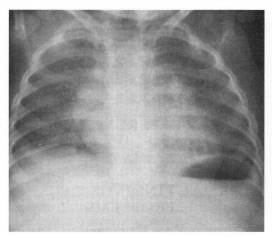 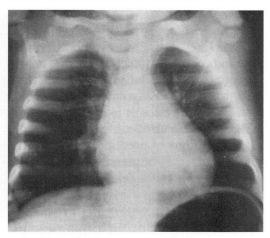

Fig. 2.144: Technical error. Expiratory view making the lungs to be appeared infiltrated and the heart enlarged with the thymus gland draped over the right cardiac silhouette.

Fig. 2.145: Technical error. Same infant (Fig. 2.144) with the deep inspiration gives a normal appearance.

Normal Lung Casting Abnormal Shadows and Causing Problems

Fallacy of Expiratory Film

In the expiratory film the lungs may appear infiltrated, heart as enlarged, and draping of thymus may appear either as hilar adenopathy or mediastinal mass.

Expiratory film (Fig. 2.144):
- Lungs appear to be infiltrated
- Heart appears to be enlarged
- Thymus gland drapes along the superior cardiac silhouette with an appearance to be hilar adenopathy or mediastinal mass.

Inspiratory Film of the Same Infant (Fig. 2.145)

- Lungs appear clear
- Heart appears to be normal in size
- Thymus is hidden in the superior mediastinum
- Diaphragm is at seventh intercostal space. Rotation of the chest may also give false appearance of infiltrates in the lung and shift of mediastinum. Normal center position to be assessed by equidistance of medial ends of clavicle from midspinal level.

Lordotic position as evidenced by the horizontal positioning of the posterior ribs is downward pointing anterior ribs may result in clustering of hilar vessels and bronchus with accentuation of vascular markings in the upper lobe.

Normal Thymus Gland

The normal thymus gland is notorious for mimicking pathology. The various radiographic appearances are:
- Covering the superior aspect of the heart like an umbrella and blends imperceptibly with the cardiac silhouette.
- Triangular in shape producing the so called "Sail Sign". This sail sign on slight rotation may mimic pneumonic consolidation of upper lobe.
- With the blending to the cardiac silhouette it may appear as mediastinal mass.

Commonly, radiographically the thymus appears up to 2–3 years of age. Normal thymus at times may be visualized up to 10–12 years of age. The picture is so altered that it may produce tumor-like superior mediastinal widening or prominence.

Blending of thymus with cardiac silhouette. Faint notch is seen at the junction of ribs (Fig. 2.146).

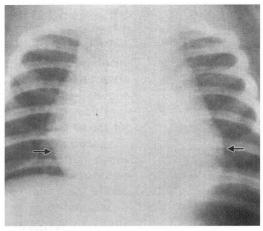

Fig. 2.146: Normal thymus notch sign. The normal thymic silhouette blends with the cardiac silhouette with a notch at its interface.

Lateral view: Normal position of the thymus in the anterior, superior mediastinal compartment with its undulating lower edge (Fig. 2.147).

❑ Pseudopneumonia appearance of thymus with its "Sail Sign" (Fig. 2.148).
❑ Rotation in another infant gives an appearance of right upper lobe pneumonia by normal thymus (Fig. 2.149).
❑ Bilaterally appearing normal thymus in the superior mediastinum giving mass-like configuration (Fig. 2.150).
❑ Large right-sided thymus obliterating cardiac silhouette with mass-like appearance (Fig. 2.151).
❑ Superior mediastinal widening due to normal thymus (Fig. 2.152).

In a 10-year-old with fever:
❑ While screening for pneumonia, suggested to be right-sided mass (Fig. 2.153).
❑ Right anterior oblique view for barium swallow showed it to be a normal thymus gland and because of that there is no pressure effect over the esophagus (Fig. 2.154).

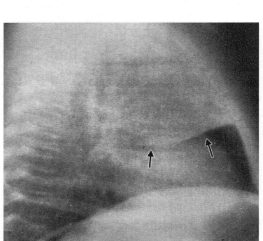

Fig. 2.147: Normal thymus. Lateral view showing normal thymus with its undulating lower edge.

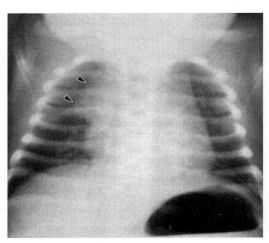

Fig. 2.148: Thymus "sail" sign. Typical sail sign of normal thymus.

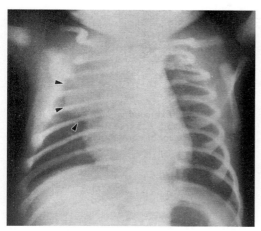

Fig. 2.149: "Pseudopneumonia sign" of normal thymus. Rotation to right causes normal thymus to appear as though a case of consolidating pneumonia of right upper lobe.

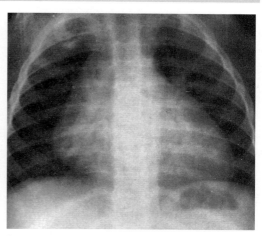

Fig. 2.151: Mass-like configuration of normal thymus gland. Large right thymic lobe suggesting a mass.

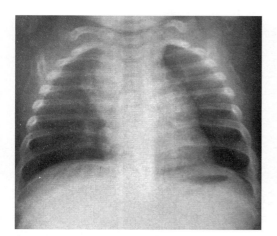

Fig. 2.150: Mass-like configuration of normal thymus gland. Bilateral superior mediastinal fullness caused by normal thymus.

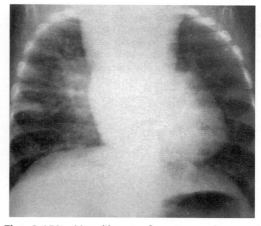

Fig. 2.152: Mass-like configuration of normal thymus gland. Peculiar superior mediastinal widening secondary to incomplete descent of normal thymus gland due to lordotic positioning.

Chest Traumas

Chest traumas whether penetrating or non-penetrating need lot of careful assessment and skillful scrutinization and vigilant survey of entire thorax. By virtue of structures like thoracic cage, cardiovascular structure, pleural space, and pulmonary parenchyma being the areas for scrutinization, a superficial careless assessment is likely to miss various important subtle findings. At the same time, the examination should be quick, careful, and thorough.

A systematic and quick screening is likely to give better results. The various structures to be scrutinized are:

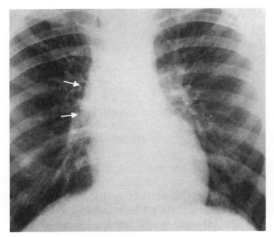

Fig. 2.153: Normal thymus in an older child. A 9-year-old child when X-ray was taken to rule out pneumonia was interpreted as a case of mediastinal mass.

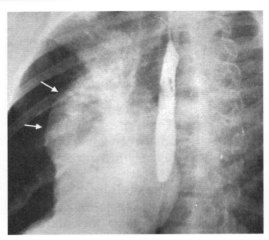

Fig. 2.154: Normal thymus in an older child. An oblique view with barium enema demonstrates the same mass was found to be normal thymus.

Thoracic Cage

❏ Subtle rib fractures are likely to be missed in the initial films
❏ Indirect evidences for subtle fractures are:
  • Subpleural hematoma
  • Pneumothorax
  • Hemothorax.
❏ Evidence for more serious intrathoracic or intra-abdominal injuries due to rib fracture is to search for by.
❏ Anterior or lateral lower thoracic rib fracture, look for splenic or liver trauma.
❏ Low posterior rib fractures—look for renal trauma.
❏ Fractures of first three ribs—search for great vessel injury and blood collections over the apex of the lung.
❏ Fractures of sternum are best visualized in lateral view.
  • Look for retro- and poststernal soft tissue injury
  • Look for cardiac injury.

Pulmonary parenchymal injuries may manifest as:

Pulmonary contusion:
❏ May manifest as pneumonia like areas of homogenous or nodular infiltrate
❏ Gets enlarged and denser in the first 24–48 hours of injury
❏ May give an appearance of mass
❏ Clears slowly.

Pulmonary hematomas:
❏ Appear like round or oval densities
❏ Resolves slowly
❏ May cavitate during the course of resolution.

Traumatic pneumatoceles:
❏ Commonly following blunt chest traumas
❏ May be seen in the pulmonary parenchyma or in the mediastinum
❏ Usually develops within minutes or hours of the injury
❏ May manifest along with other forms of pulmonary injuries
❏ May appear as round, oval, single or multiple or may contain blood
❏ Generally thin walled air cysts which may enlarge rapidly
❏ The lesion in mediastinum may appear elongated and paraspinal in position as they are located in the inferior pulmonary ligament

- Relatively innocuous
- Mostly, small slowly progressive and becomes smaller and finally disappear over 2–3 weeks period.

Catastrophic injuries to respiratory system: They are bronchial or tracheal tear or fracture and torsion of the lung.

Bronchial fracture is characterized by:
- Massive atelectasis should be presumed to be secondary to bronchial fracture until proven otherwise.
- *Massive pneumothorax:*
  - When lung is completely detached the upright view will show the lungs to fall to the bottom of the hemithorax
  - In other forms of bronchial fracture
  - The air column in the proximal portion of the fracture bronchus may appear tapered or beveled
  - The air may be seen tracking along the bronchial wall itself
  - If bleeding fluid will be seen in the hemithorax.

With tracheal tear:
- Pneumomediastinum is more common than pneumothorax
- With bleeding mediastinum appears widened.

Torsion of lung:
- Lung makes 180° turn around its hilus and so the vascular pattern of upper lobe is inverted
- With subsequent infarction radiographic diagnosis becomes difficult.

Cardiovascular manifestations of blunt chest injury:
- Bloody or serous pericardial effusion
- Myocardial contusion
- Traumatic aneurysm of heart
- Traumatic aneurysm of aorta
- Aortic or great vessel injury, radiographically may appear as progressively developing superior mediastinal widening or the collecting of blood in the apex of the left lung.

Pulmonary contusion:
- Diffuse nodular infiltrate in the right lung and more in the apex (Fig. 2.155)
  - Left pneumothorax with superimposed left apical lung contusion
- After few hours both the contused areas became more consolidated (Fig. 2.156).

Pulmonary hematoma with cavitation:
- Mass-like lesion in the right upper lobe due to hematoma (Fig. 2.157)
- A few days later a cavity developed in the hematoma (Fig. 2.158)
- More than a month, a thin walled cavity remained (Fig. 2.159).

Traumatic pneumatocele:
- Two spherical thin-walled pneumatocele in the contused left lung (Fig. 2.160)
- Large post-traumatic pneumatocele on the right (Fig. 2.161)
- Traumatic pneumatocele with air and fluid level due to blunt (Fig. 2.162).

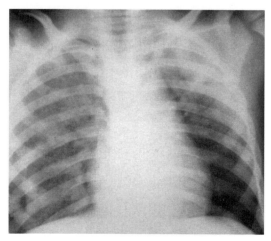

Fig. 2.155: Pulmonary contusion. Note the diffuse nodular infiltrate in the right lung and more confluent in the upper lobe. Also note the pneumothorax and lesser contusion in the left apex.

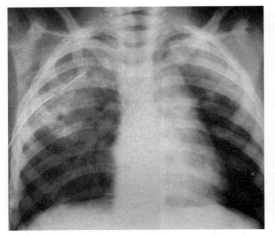

Fig. 2.156: Pulmonary hematoma with cavitation. Note a mass-like lesion in the right upper lobe.

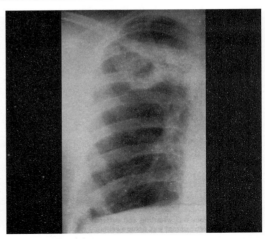

Fig. 2.158: Pulmonary hematoma with cavitation. More than a month later, a thin-walled cavity remains.

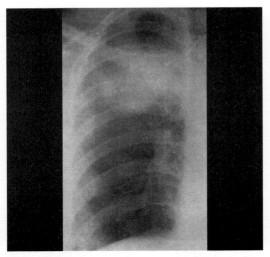

Fig. 2.157: Pulmonary hematoma with cavitation. A few days later, note that a cavity is developing in this hematoma.

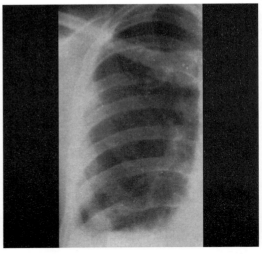

Fig. 2.159: Traumatic lung with paramediastinal pneumatocele. A thin-walled pneumatocele remained even after 1 month of injury.

Traumatic pneumatocele in inferior pulmonary ligament:

Characteristically elongated, paraspinal air collection in the inferior pulmonary ligament with air and fluid level (Figs. 2.163 and 2.164).

❑ Pneumothorax on the right
❑ Widened mediastinum
❑ Tube is in the normal position.

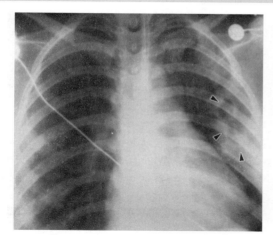

Fig. 2.160: Traumatic pneumatocele. Note two spherical thin-walled pneumatocele in the contused left lung.

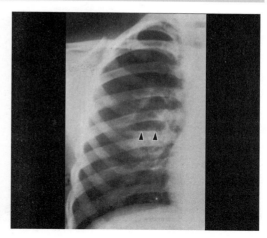

Fig. 2.162: Traumatic pneumatocele. Arrows heads—air and fluid level due to air and blood in the pneumatocele.

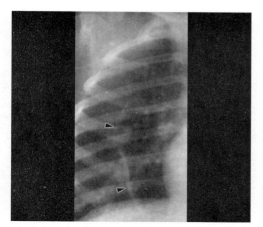

Fig. 2.161: Large post-traumatic pneumatocele on the right.

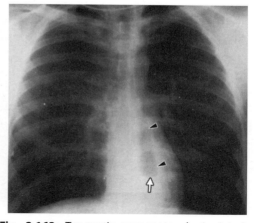

Fig. 2.163: Traumatic pneumatocele in interior pulmonary ligament. Small arrow elongated, paraspinal air collection in the inferior pulmonary ligament. Inferior arrow–air and fluid level.

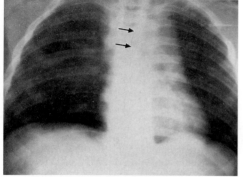

Fig. 2.164: Widened superior mediastinum and pleural fluid but no traumatic aneurysm: Pneumothorax on the right; widened mediastinum; tube is in the normal position.

▌ DIGITAL CHEST RADIOGRAPHY

Despite the advent of various modern radiological investigatory gadgets chest X-ray remains to be one of the most celebrated investigation in the nook and corner of the globe.

The main advantages of chest radiographs are:

- ❏ The speed at which they can be acquired and interpreted
- ❏ The low cost and
- ❏ The low radiation exposure.

Erect X-ray chest in day-to-day life and portable radiographs in intensive care units (ICUs) are main tools of rapid diagnostic investigations. Chest radiography is responsible for approximately 30–40% of all X-ray examinations performed, regardless of the level of health-care delivery.

There are wide attenuation differences between lungs, heart, and mediastinum in routine classical X-ray chest and fine details are likely to be missed. In such a situation digital radiography has come to rescue by its dynamic range of spatial resolution. It is able to provide accurate display of even small and focal lesion by the way of high attenuation areas such as the mediastinum and retrocardiac regions and avoiding scattering of rays. The introduction of digital radiography has revolutionized and improved image quality and allowed for further reduction of the radiation exposure of the patients.

What is Digital Radiography?

This is cassette-less and uses flat panel detectors or charge coupled devices connected to a computer.

In digital radiography digital X-ray sensors and digital image capture device are used instead of traditional film. Advantages include time efficiency and less radiation and image of similar contrast to conventional radiography can be obtained.

Some of the advanced techniques which may play an increasing role in the future are temporal subtraction, dual energy subtraction, digital tomosynthesis, and computer-aided detection (CAD) which may result in better detection and interpretation of chest X-rays. Some of the efficient services in digital radiography are its rapid production of high quality images, wide transmission of it wherever necessary and in demand, keeping it in E-file by quick archievement and retrievement.

Advantages of Digital Radiography (Figs. 2.165A and B)

- ❏ Reduced radiation dose of more than 75%.
- ❏ X-ray image enhancement by making the images darker or lighter on demand and enlarging if necessary.
- ❏ Enhanced clarity of X-ray image quality that can surpass traditional film.
- ❏ Minimal office space and maximal filing in a database and networked to access at our convenient.
- ❏ No need for harmful photographic chemical developers.
- ❏ Time efficiency by bypassing chemical processing and the ability to digitally enhance and store X-ray images and all the images are just a few clicks away.
- ❏ No more lost images as the images are automatically and immediately stored under picture archiving and communication systems (PACS).
- ❏ Quick image sharing with the help of PACS allows to get second opinion quickly and for

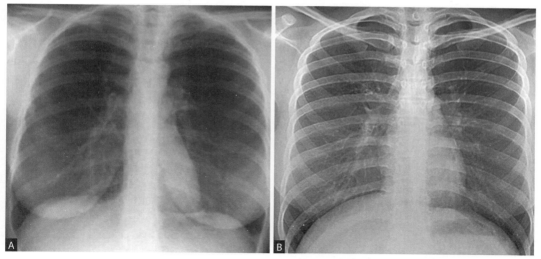

Figs. 2.165A and B: (A) Conventional X-ray chest; (B) Digital X-ray chest.

much faster diagnosis thus providing better collaboration between two professionals.

☐ Easier to use and minimal training to handle digital radiography equipment than conventional radiography.

☐ Lesser chance of artifact.

Disadvantages

☐ Cost

☐ Medicolegal: The ability to manipulate the images fraudulently to medicolegal purposes.

What is the Future of Digital Radiography?

Digital radiography is toward filmless field which needs to maintain evidence-based medicine to provide a better patient care for which in future, better detectors, faster processing, more powerful computers, bigger and sharper displays, efficient archiving may likely to transform the way the entire medical imaging is due in future.

INTERESTING CASE SCENARIOS IN X-RAY CHEST

Case 1 (Fig. 2.166)

A 25-day-old infant has presented with worsening respiratory distress and progressing apnea and cyanosis.

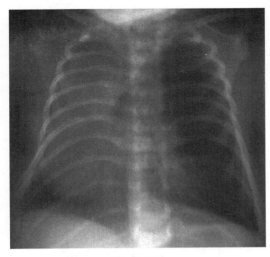

Fig. 2.166

1. Herniating left lung into the right chest.
2. Widening of ribs on the left side.
3. Mediastinal shift to the right.
4. Low placed left hemidiaphragm.
5. Atelectasis of left lower lobe.
6. Normally placed right hemidiaphragm.
7. No fluid or infiltrates.

Diagnosis: Congenital lobar emphysema of left upper lobe.

Case 2 (Fig. 2.167)

A 2-year-old child presented with a history of fever, noisy breathing, a harsh cough, and drooling.

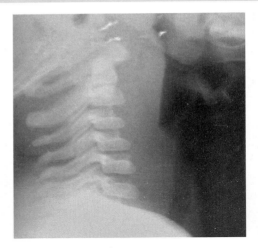

Fig. 2.167

1. The normal shaped epiglottis.
2. The preserved pre-epiglottis space.
3. The patent airway.
4. There is soft tissue swelling of prevertebral space.

Diagnosis: Retropharyngeal abscess.

Case 3 (Fig. 2.168)

A 2-year-old male child presented with acute onset of fever with rapidly progressing dysphagia, dyspnea, and drooling of saliva.

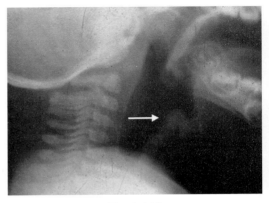

Fig. 2.168

1. Thump-like epiglottis.
2. The thickened aryepiglottic folds.
3. The preserved pre-epiglottic space to some degree.
4. The retropharyngeal space is not widened.

Diagnosis: Epiglottitis.

Case 4 (Fig. 2.169)

A 1-year-old male with barking cough and noisy breathing.

Mild degree of subglottic airway narrowing.

Diagnosis: Viral croup.

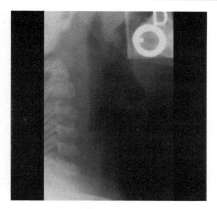

Fig. 2.169

Case 5 (Figs. 2.170A to C)

History of 1 month duration of wheezing, coughing, and rhinorrhea in a 15-month-old child.

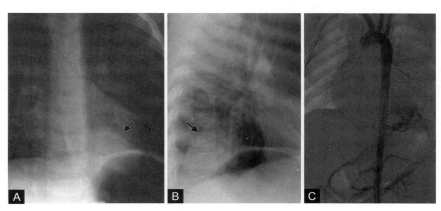

Figs. 2.170A to C

1. *Chest PA view*: A triangular density of the medial left lung base.
2. *Lateral view*: Same density is seen posteriorly over the left lung base.
3. *Contrast-injected aortogram* shows a large anomalous vessel from the infra-diaphragmatic portion of the aorta that supplies the abnormal density at the left lung base.

Diagnosis: Pulmonary sequestration.

Case 6 (Figs. 2.171A and B)

A 2-year-old child is brought to the emergency department with history of acute onset of choking which was partially relieved after some time. Looking at this X-ray, did the child ingest a battery or a coin and is it located in the esophagus or the trachea?

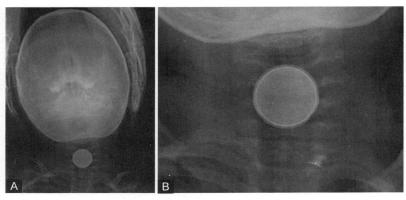

Figs. 2.171A and B

1. Battery in esophagus.
2. The child swallowed a disk battery iden-tified by the distinctive double-circle enhancement at the edge of the circular radio-opaque object. It is in the esophagus because if it were in the trachea it would project in a sagittal plane rather than the coronal plane due to the cartilages surrounding the trachea. This could be confirmed by a lateral film.

Case 7 (Fig. 2.172)

A neonate in the NICU develops an increased respiratory rate, use of accessory muscles, lower oxygen saturation, and diminished lung sounds on the right. He is intubated and a chest X-ray is ordered.

What disease pathology does the neonate have?

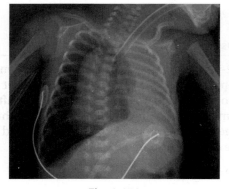

Fig. 2.172

1. Hyperlucent and hyperinflated right pleural space.
2. Collapsed and compressed right lung.
3. Shift of mediastinum to left.

Diagnosis: Right tension pneumothorax.

Case 8 (Fig. 2.173)

A 5-month-old infant with complaint of increasing respiratory distress is also pre-senting with fever and paroxysmal cough and getting worse in the past 2 days.

What does the chest X-ray reveal?

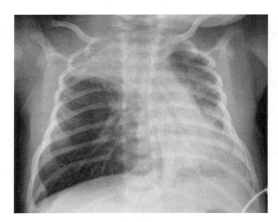

Fig. 2.173

1. Lung hyperinflation
2. Flattened diaphragm

3. Opacification in the right lung apex and left lung base from atelectasis.

Diagnosis: Bronchiolitis.

Obviously, the same changes can be seen in the X-ray of a child with acute asthma. This is one reason why children with acute asthma are often misdiagnosed as having pneumonia. Clinical correlation is very very important in arriving at correct diagnosis.

Case 9 (Fig. 2.174)

A 6-month-old infant with high fever, lethargy, refusal of feed is having rapid shallow breathing at a rate of 70 breaths/min and is presenting with rales in the right lower lung field.

What does the chest X-ray reveal?

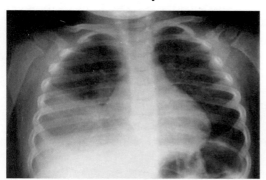

Fig. 2.174

The dense consolidation in the right lower lobe is most consistent.

Diagnosis: Bacterial pneumonia.

Case 10 (Fig. 2.175)

A 10-year-old female presented with fever, cough, breathlessness, and chest pain.

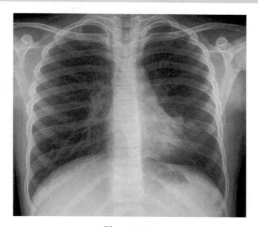

Fig. 2.175

X-ray reveals:
1. Positive silhouette of left heart border.
2. Faint opacification adjacent to the left heart border.
3. No mediastinal shift.

Diagnosis: Left lingular lobe consolidation.

After 6 weeks repeat X-ray shows normal chest (Fig. 2.176).

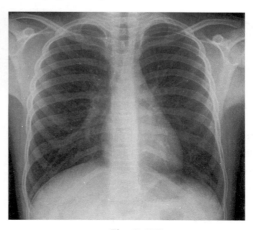

Fig. 2.176

Cardiovascular System

M Zulfikar Ahamed

■ X-RAYS GENERAL

Chest X-ray continues to have an important and integral role in the diagnosis of both congenital heart disease (CHD) and acquired heart disease (AHD) in children. Its role may have declined over the past two decades because of many factors. Technological innovations in imaging like echocardiography and magnetic resonance imaging (MRI) have contributed to noninvasively characterizing cardiac abnormalities completely. Late diagnosis of CHD has become uncommon thereby causing decline of classical X-ray appearances. Both these developments have many times obviated the need of an X-ray chest. However, conventional radiology still has a significant place in clinical cardiology as a very useful clinical tool, as it is simple, convenient, and inexpensive. It can be a fair screening tool. On many occasions, it is also useful in excluding noncardiac causes in distressed newborn or infant.

Chest X-ray is a reflection of both abnormal anatomy and abnormal hemodynamics in CHD. Chest X-rays in CHD can be occasionally diagnostic. Most often, they are useful in pointing to a diagnostic possibility. Chest X-rays are taken in three situations in pediatric cardiology:

1. Diagnostic issues in both CHD and AHD
2. Preoperative and postoperative evaluation
3. Periodic evaluation of already diagnosed heart disease.

Note: It has to be noted that a normal chest X-ray need not rule out structural heart problem and conversely a normal heart can have an apparently abnormal cardiac shadow.

Taking a Chest X-ray

In children with suspected heart lesions, X-ray chest frontal view is taken, which is most often a posteroanterior (PA) view (Fig. 3.1). Anteroposterior (AP) view is taken in small infants (Fig. 3.2). Lateral view is ordered occasionally. Contrast X-rays are limited to assessing potential vascular ring, vascular sling, or abnormality in arch of aorta. Fluoroscopy has outlived its purpose and is used

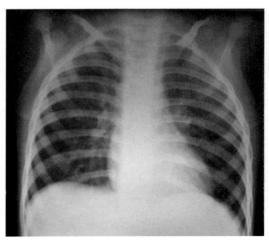

Fig. 3.1: Chest X-ray posteroanterior (PA) view. Note that heart shadow is more prominent than that of spine and ribs are more oblique.

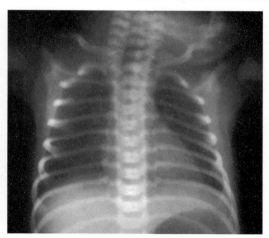

Fig. 3.2: Chest X-ray anteroposterior (AP) view. Spine is very prominent and the ribs are horizontal.

sometimes to assess prosthetic valve function. X-rays are usually taken using a nonportable machine. Portable X-rays are invariably AP (where the plate is placed on the back of the patient and X-rays are directed from front). They have an inherent limitation, creating an impression of cardiomegaly. Apart from conventional X-ray machines, digital X-ray equipment is becoming popular. Digital X-rays can be digital radiograph (DR) or computerized radiograph (CR). DR can be of indirect format or direct format.

Direct digital format are filmless. DRs have the advantages of ability for storage, archival, and transmission. There is probably less of radiation and less of time consumption. When a chest X-ray is taken, the X-ray plate is placed in front of the patient and X-rays fall from behind (PA view). AP view is obtained in a small infant. The preferable view is PA view, with the child or infant placed in the upright position.

The X-ray source-plate distance is conventionally 180 cm in adults. The distance is less in children and 100 cm in infants. The exposure time is currently less than

1/100 second, reducing motion blurring. It is taken during inspiration, which may not be always possible in infants. In a properly taken inspiratory film, the diaphragm is at the level of eighth or ninth posterior rib or sixth anterior rib.

Special Concerns in X-ray in Infants

A normal chest X-ray in an infant may not be taken in inspiration due to logistic reasons and will also contain thymic shadow, which can mimic cardiomegaly.

❑ Thymus can mimic supracardiac total anomalous pulmonary vein connection (TAPVC).
❑ Lying down may also cause apparent cardiomegaly.
❑ Over exposure of X-rays can reduce pulmonary vascular markings and under exposure, increase markings.
❑ Digital X-rays may cause slight increase in cardiac size.

Note: Newborn X-rays may be more blackish than normal and can appear oligemic. There can be apparent cardiomegaly due to horizontal position of the heart.

Heart Borders

Normally right heart border consists of right atrium below and superior vena cava (SVC) above. Occasionally ascending aorta can form part of upper right border and inferior vena cava (IVC), the lower right border. Left heart border is made up of aortic knuckle, pulmonary artery, left atrial appendage, and left ventricle (LV) from above downward (Fig. 3.3).

Lungs are divided into three zones vertically: medial, intermediate, and lateral. In the horizontal axis, lung is also divided into upper zone and lower zone. These regional divisions are mainly useful in assessing

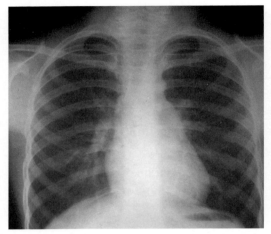

Fig. 3.3: Borders of the heart. On the right, right atrium, a portion of ascending aorta and SVC can be seen. Left heart border has a slightly prominent aortic knuckle, main pulmonary artery segment, left atrium appendage, and left ventricle shadow.

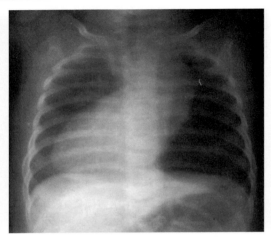

Fig. 3.4: Dextrocardia with situs solitus. Major heart shadow to the right, with apex pointing to right, liver on right and stomach shadow on left.

vascularity. Lung vascularity can be arterial (sharp and well defined) and venous (indistinct and ill defined). Both can coexist.

Reading a Chest X-ray

Whenever a chest X-ray is assessed, one must note the following items:
- Age of the child
- Date of X-ray
- Position (marker): left or right
- View: AP or PA.

Location of the Heart

Position: Situs.

Generally, the heart shadow will be predominantly on the left side with apex pointing to left.

Approximately two-third of heart shadow will be on the left half of the thorax and one-third to the right.

There can be cardiac malposition in which the heart is on the right. Malpositions can be true dextrocardia or dextroposition. Dextrocardia will have the following characteristics:
- Predominant cardiac shadow will be on the right with apex pointing to right.
- Base to apex axis is to the right.
- Generally, the diaphragm will be lower on the side of apex.

Dextrocardia can have either situs solitus—liver shadow on right and stomach shadow on left (Fig. 3.4) or situs inversus— liver shadow on left and stomach shadow on right (Fig. 3.5).

Heart can be in midline—mesocardia (Fig. 3.6). In dextroposition, the heart is on the right side due to pull or push by thoracic structures (Fig. 3.7).

Examples are as follows:
- Diaphragmatic hernia—push
- Lobar emphysema—push
- Agenesis of lung—pull
- Collapse of lung—pull.

Heart can be on the left with situs inversus levocardia with situs inversus.

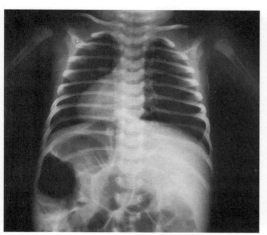

Fig. 3.5: Dextrocardia with situs inversus. Stomach shadow is to the right and liver is on the left.

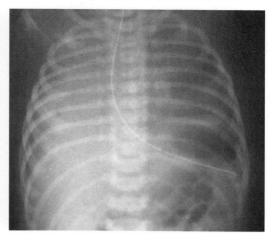

Fig. 3.7: Dextroposed heart. The cardiac shadow is on the right. However, there is crowding of ribs on the right suggesting hypoplasia of the lung pulling the heart to right.

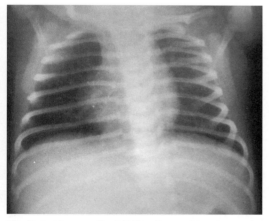

Fig. 3.6: Mesocardia. Midline heart. Liver is on the right side.

Presence of CHD in Cardiac Malposition

❏ Levocardia; situs solitus—normal arrangement, 1%
❏ Levocardia; situs inversus—100%
❏ Dextrocardia; situs solitus—90%
❏ Dextrocardia; situs inversus—5%.

Size of the Heart

Assessment of the heart size is generally subjective. However, an objective measure can be made by cardiothoracic ratio (CTR). This is derived by measuring the maximum internal thoracic diameter at the level of diaphragm and measuring maximum cardiac diameter and dividing the latter by the former.

Normal CTR in adult is 45% (mean) and in infants around 55% (mean) (Fig. 3.8). Cardiomegaly is defined as CTR more than 50% in adults, 55% in infants, and 57% in newborn. As a generalization, a CTR of more than 60% in an infant or newborn can be considered as cardiomegaly (Figs. 3.9 to 3.11).

A small heart (microcardia) is said to exist by radiograph if CTR is less than 40%. The causes are Addison's disease, severe protein energy malnutrition (PEM), anorexia nervosa, and asthma.

Contour

The contour of the heart shadow in PA view usually gives information regarding ventricular dominance (enlargement/hypertrophy).

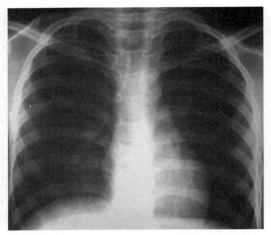

Fig. 3.8: Normal heart size. Cardiothoracic ratio is less than 50%.

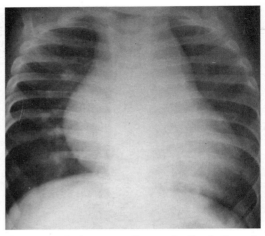

Fig. 3.10: Moderate cardiomegaly. Cardiothoracic ratio is approximately 65%.

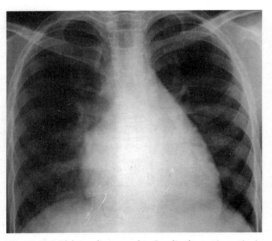

Fig. 3.9: Mild cardiomegaly. Cardiothoracic ratio is approximately 55%.

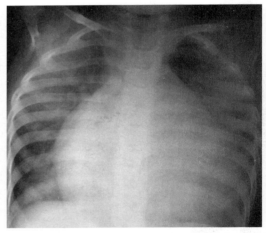

Fig. 3.11: Marked cardiomegaly. Cardiothoracic ratio is nearly 75% or more.

Normal apex is formed by LV. Mild right ventricular enlargement does not cause cardiomegaly. Modest or marked enlargement can cause cardiomegaly. This is accompanied by a rotated apex, which is laterally and upwardly displaced and elevated from diaphragm. It is called an upturned apex. An upturned apex without cardiomegaly occurs in right ventricular hypertrophy (RVH) (Fig. 3.12).

RV Apex Occurs with

No cardiomegaly:
- ☐ Tetralogy of Fallot (TOF)
- ☐ Valvular pulmonary stenosis
- ☐ Severe pulmonary artery hypertension

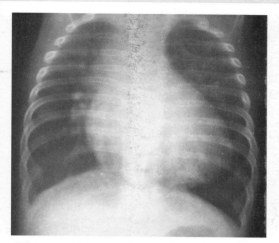

Fig. 3.12: Right ventricle apex. Note the upturned apex.

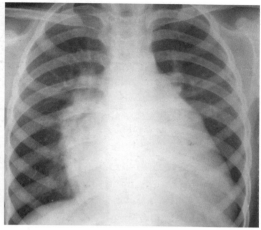

Fig. 3.13: Left ventricle apex. The apex is shifted to down and to left and sagging.

- ❏ Double outlet right ventricle (DORV), ventricular septal defect (VSD), and pulmonary stenosis (PS).

Cardiomegaly:
- ❏ d-transportation of great arteries (d-TGA)
- ❏ DORV, VSD, and pulmonary arterial hypertension (PAH)
- ❏ Atrial septal defect (ASD) with Eisenmenger syndrome
- ❏ TAPVC
- ❏ ASD
- ❏ VSD with PAH.

Left ventricle is border forming on the left side and hence can be evidently enlarged easily. The apex is shifted down and out (laterally) and sags. It can be even below the diaphragm in a radiograph. There will be rounding off the apex and elongation of long axis of LV (Fig. 3.13). In addition, in dilated cardiomyopathy (DCM), heart can be globular (Fig. 3.14).

In LV aneurysm, there could be a bulge on the left heart border. Cardiomegaly with LV apex occurs in the following:
- ❏ Patent ductus arteriosus (PDA), large shunt

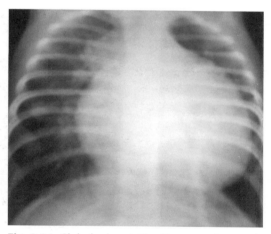

Fig. 3.14: Globular heart. Significant cardiomegaly (70%) with globularity.

- ❏ Large VSD
- ❏ Atrioventricular septal defect (AVSD) with severe mitral regurgitation (MR)
- ❏ Significant MR, aortic regurgitation (AR)
- ❏ Dilated cardiomyopathy.

Atrial Enlargement: Right Atrial Enlargement

Right atrium (RA) is border forming on the right part of heart shadow. Visible enlargement is relatively rare in children. It is evidenced by the following:

- ❐ A prominent convexity on the right side, which is lower and more lateral
- ❐ RA can be seen as a large diffuse bulge on the right side.
- ❐ The right atrial shadow/bulge will occupy at least 2.5 interspaces.
- ❐ Distance from midline to right heart border will be more than 5.5 cm in adul-WWts and more than 4.0 cm in children (Fig. 3.15).

Right atrium enlargement usually coexists with RVH. Examples are severe PS, severe PAH, DORV, d-TGA, and complete AVSD. It can be present without RVH also—Ebstein's anomaly, tricuspid atresia (TA), and right ventricle (RV) endomyocardial fibrosis (EMF).

Left Atrial Enlargement

Only left atrial appendage forms part of left heart border, just below main pulmonary artery (MPA) segment. Left atrial enlargement (LAE) can manifest in the following ways:

- ❐ Prominent left atrium (LA) appendage on left heart border (normally concave)
- ❐ Elevation of left bronchus (well appreciated in well penetrated or digital X-ray)
- ❐ Splaying of left and right bronchi with the widening of carinal angle
- ❐ "Shadow on shadow" (double shadow) appearance extending to right heart border (Fig. 3.16)
- ❐ Left atrial enlargement can occur in both CHD and AHD. It is most prominent in PDA, VSD, AVSD, MR, and mitral stenosis (MS) (Fig. 3.17).

Great Vessels

Ascending aorta can be border forming on the right side and aortic knuckle is the upper most part of left heart border. Dilated aorta—ascending or knuckle, can be found in aortic stenosis (AS), AR, coarctation and aortic aneurysm, tricuspid aortic valve with no AS, and also systemic hypertension (Fig. 3.18).

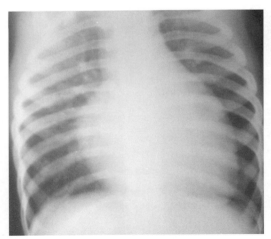

Fig. 3.15: Right atrial enlargement. Note the convex bulge on the right heart border, occupying almost four interspaces.

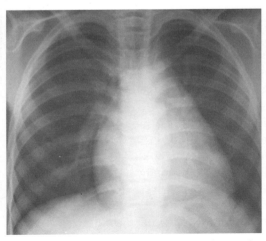

Fig. 3.16: Left atrial enlargement. Note the "straight" left heart border and "shadow on shadow" appearance.

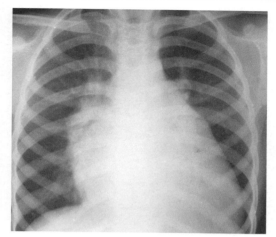

Fig. 3.17: Biatrial enlargement. Both right atrial enlargement and left atrial enlargement are present.

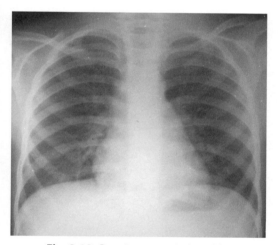

Fig. 3.18: Prominent aortic knuckle.

Arching of aorta can be usually left. Right aortic arch can be found in many CHD, especially cyanotic. Arching can be made out by ipsilateral indentation and/or deviation of trachea.

Right aortic arch in CHD:

TOF	25%
TOF, pulmonary atresia	30%
Truncus arteriosus	30–50%
d-TGA, VSD	5–10%
VSD alone	2.5%

Main pulmonary artery and its branches have to be assessed. MPA divides into right pulmonary artery (RPA) and left pulmonary artery (LPA). LPA is the continuation of MPA. RPA, shortly after origin, divides into a smaller ascending branch [right upper pulmonary artery (RUPA)] and a larger descending branch [right descending pulmonary artery (RDPA)]. In a chest X-ray, MPA, LPA, and RDPA are usually assessed. RPA is masked by cardiac shadow (Figs 3.19 and 3.20).

In adults, both LPA and RDPA are 14 mm in size near hilum. If the value is more than 15 mm, they are said to be large. Pulmonary arteries are dilated in large L-R shunts, PAH, Eisenmenger syndrome, PS, idiopathic dilatation of PA, and absent pulmonary valve syndrome.

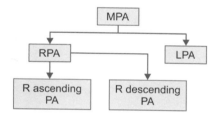

Pulmonary Vascularity

Assessment of pulmonary vascularity in suspected CHD is a major step in the diagnosis. Both acyanotic and cyanotic CHD are categorized by abnormal pulmonary vascularity. The traditional examples are L→R shunts and congenital cyanotic lesions. Vascularity of lung in both CHD and AHD can be:

❑ Normal or
❑ Abnormal.

Abnormality may be in volume, distribution, or combined.

a. Volume — Increased flow (↑PBF)
             Decreased flow (↓PBF)

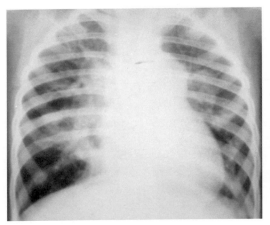

Fig. 3.19: Dilated pulmonary artery. Markedly dilated main pulmonary artery and left pulmonary artery with dilated right descending pulmonary artery can be seen. Vascularity is either normal or slightly increased.

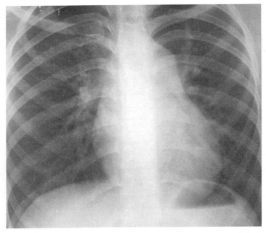

Fig. 3.20: Dilated main pulmonary artery and left pulmonary artery. Vascularity is reduced.

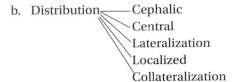

b. Distribution——Cephalic
　　　　　　　　　Central
　　　　　　　　　Lateralization
　　　　　　　　　Localized
　　　　　　　　　Collateralization

c. Combined

Note: Lung vascularity abnormality may be either arterial or venous, or both.

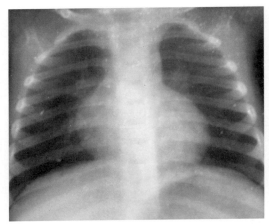

Fig. 3.21: Pulmonary oligemia. Lung vascularity is reduced. PA and branches are not at all prominent.

Generally, in evaluating CHD or AHD, we can classify pulmonary flow into four broad categories:

1. Oligemia [decreased pulmonary blood flow (PBF)]
2. Plethora (increased PBF); also called pleonemia
3. Pulmonary venous hypertension (PVH)
4. Pulmonary edema

The first two are arterial and the latter ones are venous in nature.

Pulmonary Oligemia

Vascular shadows are reduced in number and extent. They are not seen even in the intermediate lung zones. MPA, LPA, and RDPA are all small. RDPA is especially useful as normally RDPA is of the same size as right lower lobe bronchus. Pulmonary oligemia typically occurs in TOF, Critical PS, Severe PAH, etc. (Fig. 3.21).

Pulmonary Plethora

Vascular shadows are numerous. They are seen extending to lateral one-third of lung fields.

End on bronchus and corresponding artery at mid lung zones will be normally equal in size. In plethora, arterial diameter will be more and end on vessels are more in number (>5 in number per both lungs) (Fig. 3.22).

MPA, LPA, and RDPA will be large. There may be accompanying LAE or right atrial enlargement (RAE). To have plethora in a L→R shunt, shunt should be at least 1.5:1.

Pulmonary plethora occurs in L→R shunts, admixture lesions like TAPVC or Truncus, d-TGA or DORV.

Differential blood flow to lungs. It can occur in the following:

- Blalock-Taussig shunt (BT shunt)
- Waterston shunt
- RPA or LPA stenosis in CHD
- Unilateral major aortopulmonary collateral arteries (MAPCA)
- Glenn shunt (Fig. 3.23).

Pulmonary Venous Hypertension

Compared to adults, PVH is less commonly found in infants and young children. Generally, acquired heart lesions are mostly responsible for PVH. Normally upper lobe veins are less prominent than lower lobe veins due to gravity effect. In early PVH, there is equalization of the venous vascularity (Fig. 3.24).

Pulmonary venous hypertension in chest X-ray chronology: PVH occurs in chest X-ray when pulmonary vein (PV) pressure is more than 12 mm Hg.

- More than 12 mm Hg—equalization of upper and lower lobe veins
- More than 15 mm Hg—Kerley B lines appear (lateral, septal)
- Kerley A lines also appear (longer, linear lines reaching the hilum). Both represent interstitial edema.
- More than 18 mm Hg—perihilar distribution of fluid occurs
- More than 25 mm Hg—Frank pulmonary edema develops

Pulmonary venous hypertension occurs in both CHD [Cor triatriatum, obstructed TAPVC, and hypoplastic left heart syndrome (HLHS)] and AHD (MS, acute MR, acute AR, and DCM).

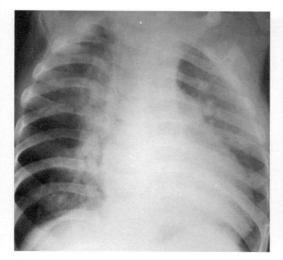

Fig. 3.22: Pulmonary plethora. Lung vascularity is increased with large number of end on vessels.

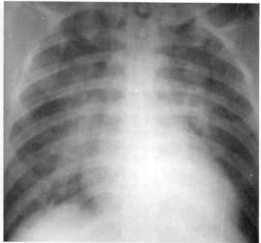

Fig. 3.23: Unequal pulmonary blood flow. Right lungs are oligemic, left is normal.

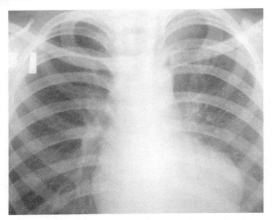

Fig. 3.24: Pulmonary venous congestion. Perihilar distribution of opacities can be seen.

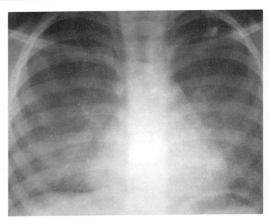

Fig. 3.25: Acute pulmonary edema. Bilateral hilar shadows, extending to periphery "Bat wing" appearance can be appreciated.

Pulmonary Edema

It occurs when pulmonary artery wedge pressure (PAWP)/PV pressure exceeds 25–28 mm Hg. There is alveolar edema, reaching to hilum giving rise to a "bat wing" appearance (Fig. 3.25).

Examples of Pulmonary Vascular Distribution Problems

❑ Cephalization—PVH

❑ Centralization—pulmonary vascular occlusive disease (PVOD)
❑ Lateralization—pulmonary embolism
❑ Localization—pulmonary AV fistula
❑ Collateralization—MAPCA in TOF.
❑ Pulmonary atresia (Table 3.1).

Other Abnormalities

Other abnormalities include cervical rib, kyphosis, scoliosis, rib notching, ductal calcium, mitral

Table 3.1: CHD and PBF.

↑PBF	↓PBF	PVH	Normal
L→R shunt	TOF	Obstr. TAPVC	PS
ASD. VSD	Tricuspid atresia	HLHS	AS
PDA	*Ebstein*	*Cor triatriatum*	Coarctation
AVSD	TGA. PS	Cong. MS	–
APW	Other TOF like CHDs	–	–
Admixture			
TAPVC. single atrium	Critical PS	–	–
DORV	–	–	–
Single ventricle	–	–	–
Truncus	–	–	–
TGA. VSD/PDA	–	–	–

(APW: Aortopulmonary window; ASD: Atrial septal defect; AVSD: Atrioventricular septal defect; DORV: Double outlet right ventricle; HLHS: hypoplastic left heart syndrome; AS: aortic stenosis; MS: mitral stenosis; PDA: Patent ductus arteriosus; PBF: Pulmonary blood flow; PS: Pulmonary stenosis; PVH: Pulmonary venous hypertension; TAPVC: Total anomalous pulmonary vein connection; TGA: Transportation of great arteries; TOF: Tetralogy of Fallot; VSD: Ventricular septal defect) and aortic valve calcium, calcification of aorta, LV aneurysm, pericardium, etc. In addition, other lung abnormalities also can coexist such as congenital diaphragmatical hernia, pneumonia, bronchiectasis, pleural effusion, and collapse.

Newborn Chest Radiograph

Chest X-ray is of less value in newborn in cardiac diagnosis, as there is not enough time to develop classical radiological findings. Lungs in the newborn may appear oligemic. One major use of X-ray is to help differentiate a cardiac pathology from lung pathology. It is also useful in diagnosing cardiac malpositions in the newborn. A standard format for cardiovascular system. X-ray reading is given in Table 3.2.

■ X-RAYS SPECIFIC

Chest Radiograph: Individual Lesions

Left-to-Right Shunts

Left-to-right shunts are divided into the following:

☐ Pretricuspid: ASD
  • Partial anomalous
  • Venous drainage (Table 3.3).

☐ Posttricuspid: VSD, PDA, aortopulmonary window (AP window), and AV septal defect

Radiology of these lesions essentially reflects hemodynamic state and is dependent on the following:

☐ Pretricuspid or posttricuspid nature
☐ Size of the defect and shunt
☐ Presence of PAH.

Atrial Septal Defect

Atrial septal defect can be ostium secundum (70%), ostium primum (20%), and sinus venosus (10%). The radiologic abnormalities are to some extent distinctive but not diagnostic.

Small ASD

There is no cardiomegaly. There may not be appreciable increase in vascularity. PA may be mildly prominent.

Moderate ASD

There is usually cardiomegaly with RV apex (upturned). Approximately 10–15% of ASD with significant L→R shunt may have a normal heart size. RAE is usual. PBF is increased with large PA and branches. RDPA

Table 3.2: Standard format for X-ray chest reading.

- Chest X-ray frontal/PA/AP
- Levocardia/Dextrocardia/Mesocardia with Situs
- Cardiomegaly—mild/moderate/marked/CT ratio
- LV contour/RV contour/can't say
- LA enlargement/RA enlargement/biatrial
- Aorta/pulmonary artery and branches
- Pulmonary vascularity/categorization
- Others—lungs, ribs, thymus, etc.
- Classic descriptions if any, e.g. figure of 8; egg on side

(AP: anteroposterior; PA: posteroanterior; LV: left ventricle; RV: right ventricle; LA: left atrium; RA: right atrium)

Table 3.3: Pretricuspid vs. posttricuspid shunt.

Radiological features	Pretricuspid shunt	Posttricuspid shunt
Cardiac size	Variable	Variable
Apex	RV	LV usually
RAE	Present	Not usual
LAE	Absent	Present
PBF	Increased	Increased
PVH	Absent	May be present
Aortic shadow	Small	Normal/large

(LAE: left atrial enlargement; LV: left ventricle; PBF: PBF: pulmonary blood flow; PVH: pulmonary venous hypertension; RV: right ventricle; RAE: right atrial enlargement) may be more prominent than LPA. There is no LA enlargement. Aorta is relatively inconspicuous (Fig. 3.26).

Large ASD

Similar findings may be noted with all the features being more prominent.

ASD with PVOD

The cardiomegaly will remain. Proximal PA and branches (MPA, LPA, and RDPA) are hugely dilated with peripheral pruning. RV apex is very prominent with significant RA enlargement.

Sinus Venosus ASD

It is similar to a moderate ASD. SVC shadow will be more prominent.

ASD with LA Enlargement

It can occur in the following:
- ❏ Adult ASD
- ❏ Atrial fibrillation
- ❏ Associated mitral valve disease.

Atrioventricular Septal Defect

Atrioventricular septal defect can occur in four different forms. Simplest is the ostium primum ASD with cleft mitral valve. Others are transitional AVSD, intermediate AVSD, and complete AVSD. Chest X-ray will show cardiomegaly invariably with increased pulmonary vascularity. Whenever there is a VSD, apex is likely to be LV type with some PVH in lung fields. There is most often biatrial enlargement except in ostium primum ASD. LV to RA shunt in AVSD can further accentuate RAE (Fig. 3.27).

Ventricular Septal Defect

Ventricular septal defect can be perimembranous (70%), muscular (20%), inlet (5–8%), and subpulmonic (<5%). They can be small, medium, large, and unrestrictive. Radiologic findings are not diagnostic but useful.

Small VSD

There is no cardiomegaly. Pulmonary vascularity is normal. PA and major branches are normal.

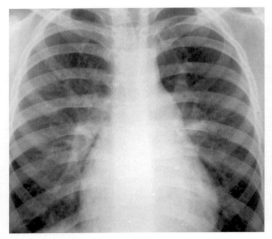

Fig. 3.26: Atrial septal defect. Note the mild cardiomegaly, right atrial enlargement, prominent PA, and increased pulmonary flow.

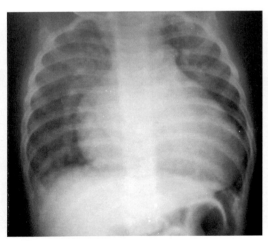

Fig. 3.27: AVSD. Cardiomegaly, biatrial enlargement, prominent pulmonary vascularity. There are no typical findings.

Moderate VSD

There is cardiomegaly of moderate degree (<60%). There is LV apex with LA enlargement. PAs are large with increased pulmonary vascularity. PVH can be superimposed on the lung vascularity indicating elevated left filling pressures. Aorta is normal in size.

Large VSD

There is significant cardiomegaly with large LA. RAE also can be present in the presence of PAH. Apex can be RV (upturned) even though usually it is LV type. Pulmonary vascularity is markedly increased with coexisting PVH. There can be patchy opacities in the lungs. Aorta is normal (Fig. 3.28).

Large VSD, PVOD

There is no or minimal cardiomegaly with RV apex. MPA and branches are large with peripheral pruning. LA enlargement may persist.

VSD with AR

Cardiomegaly with LV apex is the norm. Aorta can be enlarged. VSD can have right aortic arch in 2.5%.

Patent Ductus Arteriosus

Patent ductus arteriosus represents 7% of all CHD. This can be trivial, small, moderate, or large.

Small PDA

No cardiomegaly is appreciable. PBF is normal. MPA and LPA may be mildly prominent.

Moderate PDA

Cardiomegaly is invariable with a distinct LV apex. There is LA enlargement with no RA enlargement. Pulmonary vascularity is increased. MPA and LPA are particularly large. Aorta is prominent (Fig. 3.29).

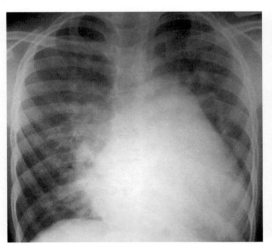

Fig. 3.28: Ventricular septal defect. Cardiomegaly, left ventricle apex, left atrial enlargement, and increased pulmonary vascularity. Main pulmonary artery and left pulmonary artery are large. There is some pulmonary venous hypertension also.

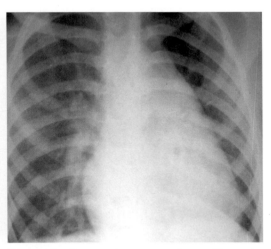

Fig. 3.29: Patent ductus arteriosus. Note the cardiomegaly with left ventricle apex, prominent left atrial enlargement, and increased pulmonary vascularity. Right atrial enlargement is not seen.

Large PDA

This will have a bigger heart with LV apex and very prominent MPA and LPA. PVH is usual, superimposed on increased PBF. Biatrial enlargement could be present.

PDA-PVOD

There is no cardiomegaly. LA enlargement may persist. PA and branches are very large with pruning of periphery. Ductal calcium can be found in adults. The clinical features of ASD, VSD, and PDA are shown in Table 3.4.

Pulmonary Stenosis

This represents 5–7% CHD; 90% are valvar.

Mild-Moderate PS

There is no cardiomegaly. RV apex can be found. RA enlargement may occur. LA is inconspicuous. Pulmonary blood flow is characteristically normal as the entire RV output goes to the lungs without diversion. PA dilatation (MPA and LPA) can be present in 80–90% of cases (Fig. 3.30).
Note: Poststenotic dilatation is not found in dysplastic pulmonary valve, infundibular PS, and in infants.

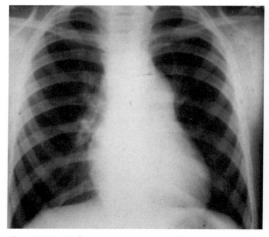

Fig. 3.30: Pulmonary stenosis. Note no cardiomegaly, poststenotic dilatation and normal lung vascularity.

Severe PS

Minimal or no cardiomegaly with prominent RV apex is seen. PBF is near normal. There is significant poststenotic dilatation (Table 3.5).

Severe PS with RV Dysfunction

In such cases, there is significant cardiomegaly with prominent RA and RV apex. Poststenotic dilatation remains. Pulmonary vascularity is diminished markedly.

Table 3.4: CXR of L→R shunt.			
	ASD	*VSD*	*PDA*
Cardiomegaly	Common	Common	Common
Apex	RV	LV or RV	LV
RAE	Present	May be present	Not usual
LAE	Absent	Present	Prominent
PBF	Increased	Increased	Increased
PVH	Absent	May be present	May be present
Aorta	Less prominent	Normal	Prominent
Pulmonary arteries	Large	Large	Larger

(ASD: atrial septal defect; LAE: left atrial enlargement; LV: left ventricle; PBF: pulmonary blood flow; PDA: patent ductus arteriosus; PVH: pulmonary venous hypertension; RAE: right atrial enlargement; RV: right ventricle; VSD: ventricular septal defect)

Table 3.5: Difference between pink TOF and severe PS.

Clinical features	Pink TOF	Mod-severe PS
Cardiac size	Normal	Normal/minimal CE
Apex	Upturned	Upturned
RAE	Absent	Present
Pulmonary artery	Concavity	Poststenotic dilatation
Arch or aorta	25% Rt	Left arch
Pulmonary vascularity	Oligemia	Normal

(PS: pulmonary stenosis; RAE: right atrial enlargement; TOF: tetralogy of Fallot)

Note: In significant valvular PS, there can be a minor inequality in blood flow. Right lung flow could be slightly less than left lung flow (Fig. 3.31).

Aortic Stenosis

It represents 5–7% of all CHD; 90% are valvular.

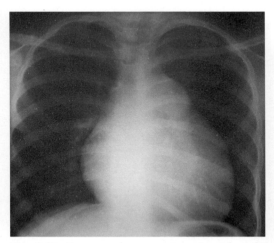

Fig. 3.31: Severe pulmonary stenosis with right ventricle dysfunction. Cardiomegaly, hugely dilated main pulmonary artery and left pulmonary artery, less prominent right pulmonary artery, and pulmonary oligemia.

Infant with Severe AS

Radiological behavior is totally different from that of a child or adolescent. There will be invariably cardiomegaly with LV apex. Significant PVH is seen in 50%. Aorta may or may not be prominent (Fig. 3.32).

Child with Severe AS

There is no or minimal cardiomegaly. LV configuration is striking. Aorta is prominent. Dilatation of aorta need not be proportional to severity of AS. LAE can be occasionally noted in severe AS.

Child with Severe AS and LV Dysfunction

Cardiomegaly is invariable. There is LAE. PVH is usual. Aorta is prominent. AS with cardiomegaly could mean the following:
- ❑ Associated AR
- ❑ Left ventricle dysfunction
- ❑ Mitral valve disease
- ❑ Secondary EFE.

Coarctation of Aorta

It represents 5% of all CHD. It is mostly postsubclavian and discrete. Behavior of

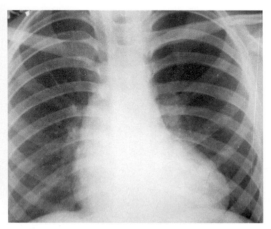

Fig. 3.32: Aortic stenosis. Note the minimal cardiomegaly, left ventricle apex, and a very prominent ascending aorta. Vascularity is normal.

coarctation of aorta (CoA) in infancy differs from that in childhood and adult.

Infant with Significant CoA

Most of the infants are present in CHF and will have cardiomegaly. The apex could be of RV type. PAs are prominent due to significant PAH. Pulmonary vascularity is normal except when there is an additional L-R shunt. Examples include VSD or PDA. PVH is usual.

Child with Significant CoA

Cardiomegaly may be minimal. Apex is LV type with the normal lung vascularity. Aorta is prominent. The characteristic findings on Chest X-ray are (Fig. 3.33) as follows:

❑ 3 sign: Due to dilatation of aorta and subclavian artery proximal to CoA and post-stenotic dilatation of descending aorta
❑ E sign on barium swallow (seldom done)
❑ Bilateral rib notching: Rib notching is evident only beyond 4–6 years. They are found in third to eighth ribs, posteriorly

due to dilatation of posterior intercostal arteries. Rib notching is a function of age. Between 6 and 40 years, the incidence is 50%. Beyond 20 years, the incidence is 75–90%.

Note: Unilateral rib notching can occur in CoA if one subclavian artery is distal to the CoA, for example, aberrant right subclavian artery.

Hypoplastic Left Heart Syndrome

This has a nondiagnostic X-ray in newborn. Cardiac size may be normal or enlarged with severe PVH. The X-ray may mimic hyaline membrane disease (HMD), especially if ASD is small. Significant RA enlargement can be seen.

Anomalous Left Coronary Artery from Pulmonary Artery

There is no characteristic radiological finding but there may be severe cardiomegaly simulating DCM (Fig. 3.34).

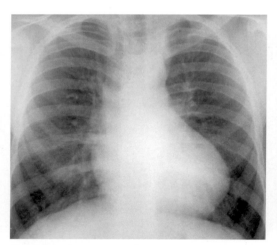

Fig. 3.33: Coarctation of aorta. No cardiomegaly, "3" appearance of aorta and rib notching which are more prominent on the left.

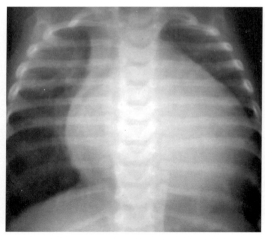

Fig. 3.34: X-ray of anomalies left coronary artery from pulmonary artery. Nothing is specific. Note the marked cardiomegaly simulating dilated cardiomyopathy.

Cyanotic Congenital Heart Disease

Cyanotic congenital heart disease (CCHD) can have either an increased PBF or decreased PBF. Occasionally, CCHD presents with PVH.

❏ CCHD with decreased PBF:
- TOF with pulmonary atresia
- TA
- TGA-VSD-PS
- AVSD-PS
- Single ventricle PS
- Truncus-PS
- DORV-VSD-PS
- L-TGA-VSD-PS
- Critical PS with ASD
- Ebstein's anomaly
- Eisenmenger syndrome.

❏ CCHD with increased PBF:
- d-TGA-IVS-VSD or PDA
- TAPVC single atrium
- DORV with single ventricle
- Truncus
- Pulmonary atresia with extensive MAPCA.

❏ CCHD with PVH:
- HLHS
- Obstructed TAPVC.

Tetralogy of Fallot

The most common CCHD and is approximately 10% of all CHD. It has characteristic X-ray findings (Fig. 3.35).

❏ There is no cardiomegaly with upturned apex
❏ Concave pulmonary bay, with small PAS
❏ Reduced pulmonary vascularity
❏ Right aortic arch in 25%
❏ "Coeur en Sabot" appearance is quite distinct
❏ The appearance may mimic a "golf club."

In a pink TOF, X-ray may look deceptively normal or even has mild cardiomegaly. Pulmonary vascularity may be normal. Normal or increased vascularity could be found in extensive MAPCA in pulmonary atresia. A lacy and reticular pattern is found on both lung fields (Table 3.6).

Cardiomegaly is quite unusual in TOF. It can be found in the presence of the following:

❏ MAPCA
❏ Restrictive VSD
❏ Infective endocarditis
❏ Anemia
❏ Associated systemic hypertension in adult
❏ Postoperative TOF with pulmonary regurgitation (PR).

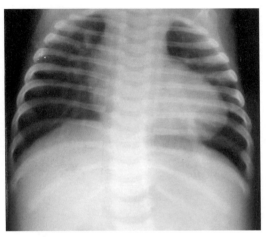

Fig. 3.35: Tetralogy of Fallot. Note minimal cardiac enlargement, right ventricle apex, no right atrial enlargement, and presence of oligemia of lungs. The wide base may be due to right arch.

Table 3.6: Differences between TOF and TA.

	TOF	TA
Cardiomegaly	None	None or minimal
Apex	RV	LV
RAE	Absent	Present and distinct
Pulmonary bay	Present	Present
Rt arch	25%	Rare
PBF	Reduced	Reduced

(LV: left ventricle; PBF: pulmonary blood flow; RV: right ventricle; RAE: right atrial enlargement; TA: tricuspid atresia; TOF: tetralogy of Fallot)

Transposition of Great Arteries

It accounts for 5% of all CHD and is the leading CCHD in the newborn. CXR appearance may be normal up to 1 week. The classical picture develops quite late, may be around 2–3 weeks.

TGA-IVS

☐ Mild cardiomegaly
☐ RV apex
☐ Right atrial enlargement
☐ Increased pulmonary vascularity (70%)
☐ Absent thymus/narrow pedicle.

Thymic absence is seen noticed beyond the second day. Posteriorly placed pulmonary artery also contributes to narrow pedicle. Right arch is rare (4%). The classic egg on side appearance is found only in 30–50% of cases (Fig. 3.36). Earlier the diagnosis, less likely it is to have classical look. There could be slightly more vascularity of right lung due to preferential flow of blood from LV to RPA.

TGA-VSD

Cardiomegaly is prominent with significant increase in pulmonary vascularity. PAs may appear large with LAE also. Right arch is found in 5–10% (Figs. 3.37 and 3.38).

Tricuspid Atresia

Tricuspid atresia accounts for 2.5% of CHD. It has a distinctive X-ray appearance (Fig. 3.39).
☐ Cardiomegaly is minimal
☐ RA enlargement is very prominent
☐ Heart can be globular with concavity on left upper border
☐ Pulmonary vascularity is diminished in 80%.

In TA with TGA, cardiomegaly and increased PBF is usual due to increased blood flow to lungs. Narrow pedicle also could be found as in regular d-TGA.

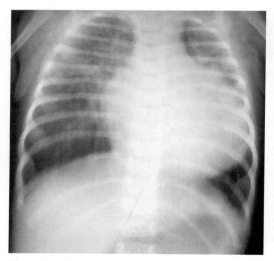

Fig. 3.36: Transportation of great arteries. Note the cardiomegaly, right ventricle apex, right atrial enlargement, narrow base, and marked increase in lung vascularity. The "egg on side" appearance with lung oligemia can be seen.

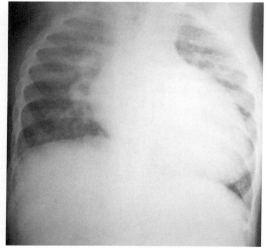

Fig. 3.37: Transposition of great arteries, ventricular septal defect and pulmonary arterial hypertension. It has a left ventricle apex which sags and huge cardiac enlargement.

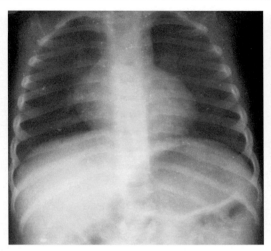

Fig. 3.38: Transposition of great arteries, ventricular septal defect, and pulmonary stenosis. The "egg on side" appearance with lung oligemia can be seen.

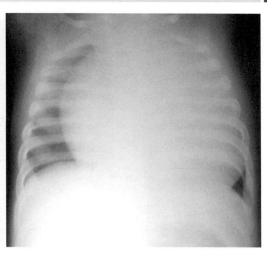

Fig. 3.40: Ebstein's anomaly. Gross cardiomegaly, ballooned right atrium and hardly any lung shadow is seen.

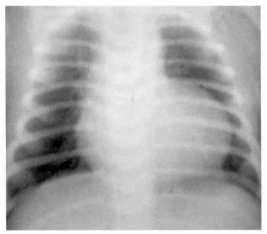

Fig. 3.39: Tricuspid atresia. Mild cardiomegaly, a square apex, right atrial enlargement, and concave pulmonary bay with oligemia.

Ebstein's Anomaly

It is a rare, but distinct CHD with characteristic X-ray findings. The characteristic appearance is massive cardiomegaly with pulmonary oligemia.

Newborn: Significant Ebstein's Anomaly

Large heart with very much enlarged RA is found with reduced pulmonary vascularity. The heart may occupy more than 80% of thoracic diameter.

Infant or Child with Ebstein's Anomaly

It represents variable cardiomegaly, depending on the severity of displacement of the valve. The features are as follows (Figs. 3.40 and 3.41):

❏ Massive cardiomegaly
❏ Dilated right ventricular outflow tract (RVOT) with a box-shaped heart
❏ Narrow pedicle
❏ Huge RA
❏ Reduced pulmonary vascularity.
  • Pulmonary vascularity depends on the presence of cyanosis. Cyanotic Ebstein's anomaly will have oligemia. Narrow base is due to non-border forming of pulmonary artery and small aorta. It may mimic pericardial effusion.

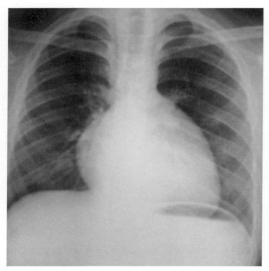

Fig. 3.41: Ebstein anomaly. Modest Cardiomegaly, right atrial enlargement and narrow base are seen. Pulmonary oligemia is evident.

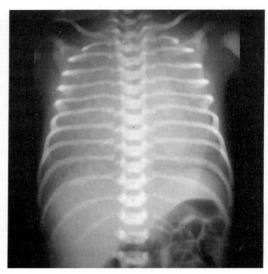

Fig. 3.42: Total anomalous pulmonary vein connection obstructed. Showing a "white washed" lung.

The important radiological differential diagnoses of severe Ebstein's anomaly are:

❒ Critical PS with RV dysfunction and reversal of flow
❒ Right ventricle EMF
❒ Pericardial effusion.

Total Anomalous Pulmonary Venous Connection

Total anomalous pulmonary vein connection can be obstructed or nonobstructed.

Obstructed TAPVC in Newborn

Cardiomegaly is unusual. There is severe PVH and pulmonary edema producing a ground glass appearance of lung fields (Fig. 3.42). It may mimic HMD. The differentiating "soft" points in HMD are as follows:

❒ Absolutely normal sized heart
❒ Air bronchogram
❒ Obliteration of heart border.

Nonobstructed TAPVC (Supracardiac)

There is significant cardiomegaly with dilated PAs and increased vascularity. RA enlargement is usual with a small aorta. The typical "figure of 8" appearance takes time to develop (3–6 months). The upper part of 8 is formed by SVC on right and vertical vein on left. The lower half is formed by RA on right and LV on left. The typical appearance is usually limited to TAPVC draining to left innominate vein (Fig. 3.43). Thymic enlargement can mimic "figure of 8" appearance (Fig. 3.44).

Scimitar syndrome is characterized by dextroposed heart, hypoplasia of right lung causing reduced lung volume, and abnormal vertical vein running on right side from down below.

Double Outlet Right Ventricle

Double outlet right ventricle can be present either with PAH (increased PBF) or PS

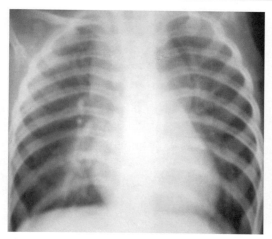

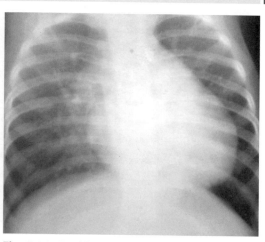

Fig. 3.43: Total anomalous pulmonary vein connection unobstructed and supracardiac. Classical "figure of 8" appearance can be seen.

Fig. 3.45: Double outlet right ventricle with pulmonary arterial hypertension. Almost like an X-ray of ventricular septal defect with right ventricle apex. Not specific.

anomaly, the X-ray may look like that of d-TGA (Fig. 3.45).

Single Ventricle

Cardiac malposition will be more common with SV. Right isomerism can coexist. SV can have PS or PAH and X-ray findings will differ accordingly LV apex could be found as most of SV are double inlet into left ventricle (DILV). Straight left heart border can occur sometimes in SV with rudimentary RV on left heart border.

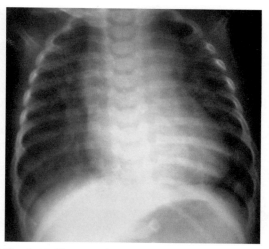

Fig. 3.44: Thymus. Thymic enlargement can mimic "figure of 8" appearance.

L-Transposition of Great Arteries

L-TGA could be found in dextrocardia with situs solitus. Hemodynamics will determine the following radiological findings:

(decreased PBF). There are no diagnostic findings. X-ray of DORV-VSD-PS will look like that of TOF with borderline cardiomegaly. DORV with PAH may look like a large VSD with PAH on X-ray with cardiomegaly, RV apex, biatrial enlargement, and increased pulmonary vascularity. In Taussig-Bing

❏ L-TGA with VSD-PS—TOF like
❏ L-TGA with VSD—VSD like.

Distinct features are ascending aortic shadow on left upper heart border due to L-posed aorta and cause straight left heart border. Cardiac enlargement could occur in the presence of the following:

❑ VSD with PAH
❑ Left AV valve regurgitation.

Truncus Arteriosus

Cardiomegaly is the rule. There is LAE and increased pulmonary vascularity. PVH is also associated. PAs are not well delineated as the MPA and branches are posteriorly placed. Arch of aorta is toward right in 30–50%. Pedicle is narrow because there is only one arterial trunk.

Note: CCHD with increased PBF—right Arch-Truncus

CCHD with decreased PBF—right Arch-TOF.

Increased lung vascularity with less well-delineated MPA and branches can be found in the following:

❑ Truncus
❑ TOF with MAPCA
❑ d-TGA with IVS.

Eisenmenger Syndrome

The standard radiological features include no or minimal cardiomegaly, RV apex, possible RAE hugely dilated proximal PAS, and peripheral pruning (Figs. 3.46 and 3.47 and Table 3.7).

Cardiac Malpositions

Dextroposed Heart

It indicates "no true dextrocardia." Heart is either pushed by congenital diaphragmatic hernia (CDH), pneumothorax, pleural effusion, emphysema, or a mass or pulled by agenesis, collapse, and fibrosis. Dextroposed

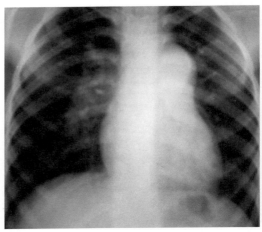

Fig. 3.46: Eisenmenger syndrome. No cardiomegaly, huge PAs, and pruning of pulmonary vessels at periphery.

Table 3.7: Eisenmenger complex.			
	ASD	*VSD/APW*	*PDA*
Cardiomegaly	Present	Absent	Absent
Apex	RV	RV	RV
Proximal pulmonary arteries	Huge	Large	Large
Pruning	Present	Present	Present
RAE	Prominent	Present	Present
Aorta	Small	Normal	Prominent
Others	–	–	Ductal Ca++

(APW: Aortopulmonary window; ASD: atrial septal defect; PDA: patent ductus arteriosus; RAE: right atrial enlargement; RV: right ventricle; VSD: ventricular septal defect)

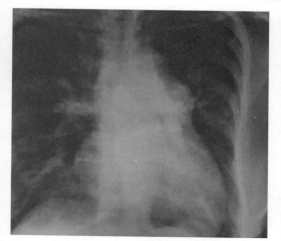

Fig. 3.47: ASD with Eisenmenger. There is cardiomegaly, prominent MPA, LPA and RPA. Right atrial enlargement and peripheral pruning of pulmonary vessels seen.

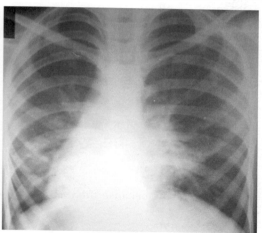

Fig. 3.48: Dextrocardia, situs inversus. It could be a Kartagener syndrome.

heart is found in scimitar syndrome, which is associated with hemi anomalous pulmonary venous connection (HAPVC).

True Dextrocardia

It can have the following:
❑ Situs solitus
❑ Situs inversus (Fig. 3.48).
   Figure 3.49 shows PDA device closure.

Levocardia with Situs Inversus

It can occur with complex CHD, especially L-TGA (Fig. 3.50).

Rheumatic Heart Diseases

Mitral Stenosis

There is no cardiomegaly. LV apex is found. LA enlargement is prominent with PVH.

   PA enlargement also could be found, due to PAH. RAE is seen only severe PAH with TR (Fig. 3.51).

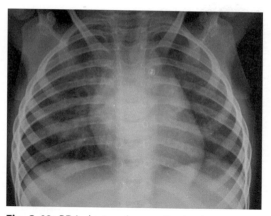

Fig. 3.49: PDA device closure. Device is seen near MPA location.

Mitral Regurgitation

It will have variable cardiomegaly with LAE. PVH and PAH occurs late in the natural history (Figs. 3.52 to 3.55). PVH in severe MR can occur in the following:
❑ LV dysfunction
❑ Acute MR
❑ Associated DCM or anomalies left coronary artery from pulmonary artery (ALCAPA).

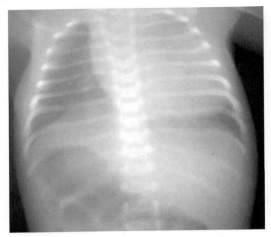

Fig. 3.50: Levocardia; situs inversus. It is extremely rare. About 99% have complex congenital heart disease. Cardiomegaly percentage in newborn, infants, and children.

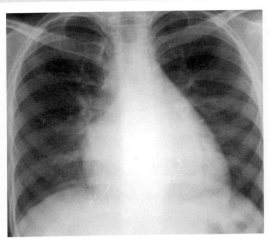

Fig. 3.52: Mitral regurgitation. Mild cardiomegaly, left atrial enlargement, and mild pulmonary venous hypertension.

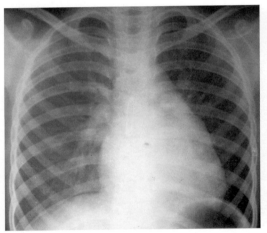

Fig. 3.51: Mitral stenosis. No cardiomegaly, left atrial enlargement and pulmonary venous hypertension.

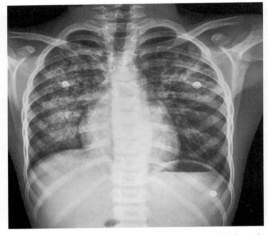

Fig. 3.53: Acute pulmonary edema in a child with acute MR. There is no cardiomegaly. Bilateral reticular appearance, more near hilum.

Aortic Regurgitation

It indicates cardiomegaly with LV Apex. Huge cardiac enlargement can occur with prominent aorta. LA enlargement is found in presence of mitral valve involvement or LV dysfunction (*See* Fig. 3.54).

Hypertrophic Cardiomyopathy

X-ray in HCM may be deceptively normal with no cardiomegaly. Occasionally mild PVH is noticeable.

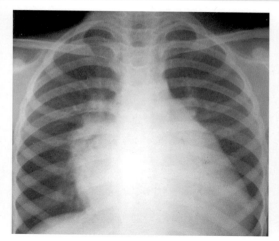

Fig. 3.54: Bivalvular rheumatic heart disease. Marked cardiac enlargement, left ventricle apex, biatrial enlargement, and pulmonary arterial hypertension.

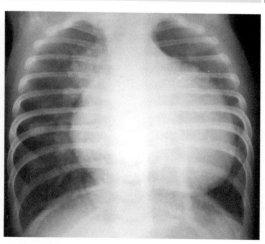

Fig. 3.56: Globular enlargement of heart. Cardiophrenic angles are intact, indicating that there is no effusion.

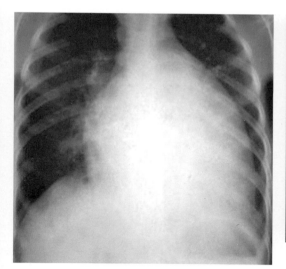

Fig. 3.55: Severe mitral regurgitation. Note huge cardiomegaly and left atrial enlargement.

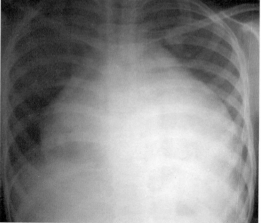

Fig. 3.57: Pericardial effusion. Huge heart, obliteration of cardiophrenic angles, and narrow base.

Dilated Cardiomyopathy

It will have cardiomegaly with globular heart and LV apex. LAE is invariable RAE occurs late, in PAH. Pleural effusion could occur (Fig. 3.56).

Pericardial Effusion

This will be characterized by the following (Fig. 3.57):
❏ Cardiomegaly with globular heart
❏ Narrow base.
❏ Sagging lower heart borders with obliteration of cardiophrenic angles

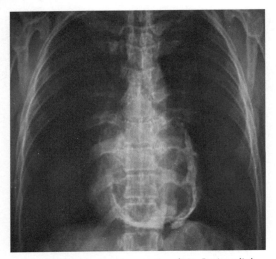

Fig. 3.58: Constrictive pericarditis. Pericardial calcification with no cardiomegaly.

❏ Stenciled out distinct cardiac margins
❏ Normal or reduced lung vascularity.

Figure 3.58 shows constrictive pericarditis and pericardial calcification with no cardiomegaly.

Note: All the abbreviations are given in Preliminary pages on Pg nos. xix and xx.

Bone and Metabolic Diseases

G Vijayalakshmi

■ INTRODUCTION

The first X-ray ever taken was that of bones. Next to the chest, the largest number of X-ray taken now is that of bones. In spite of so many advancements in the field of imaging, X-ray is and will remain the mainstay in diagnosis of skeletal pathology. There are certain features in bone peculiar to children. After fusion of epiphysis, the mature adult bone is a continuous mass. However, there are five radiologically distinct parts in a growing bone. They are the epiphysis, metaphysis and diaphysis, physis, and zone of provisional calcification. An epiphysis is present at each end of the long limb bones, but is found at only one end of the metacarpals (at proximal end in first and distal end in second to fifth metacarpals), metatarsals (proximal in first and distal in second to fifth metatarsals), phalanges (proximal ends), clavicles, and ribs. In contrast to long bones, flat or membranous bones do not have a single growth plate, but many epiphyses are placed at intervals circumferentially. The slightly expanded portion at the end of the diaphysis is the metaphysis. In between the epiphysis and the metaphysis is a lucent layer, the physis, or growth plate (Fig. 4.1). In between the physis and the metaphysis is a white line, which is the zone of provisional cartilage. The physis is composed of innumerable cartilage cells that have an amazing potential for multiplication. The cartilage cells near the epiphysis proliferate, undergo hypertrophy, and move to the metaphyseal side. Here they die and get calcified. This is the zone of provisional calcification, consisting of dead and calcified cartilage cells. It is then invaded by osteoclasts, which resorb the calcified cartilage. Osteoclasts are followed by osteoblasts. Osteoblasts lay down osteoid, which is then mineralized. Both calcification of cartilage and mineralization of osteoid are affected in vitamin D deficiency. Between the ages of 18 years and 25 years, the cartilage cells gradually cease to proliferate, the epiphyseal plates close, fade, and leave a thin

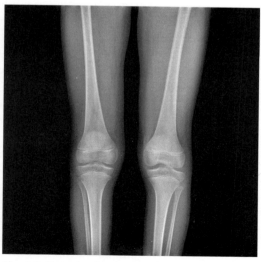

Fig. 4.1: Note the thin lucent physis in between the epiphysis and metaphysis in this 9-year-old child.

white line. This signifies that bone growth has stopped. It has been found that the fastest growing bone ends are the distal femur, proximal tibia, distal radius, and proximal humerus. The clavicle is the last bone to stop growing. The aforementioned sequence results in linear growth of bone. Thickness of bone is achieved by osteoblasts derived from the periosteum. Increase in thickness goes on even after linear growth ceases. Long bones have a tubular shaft composed of solid bone tissue enclosing a cavity. The medullary cavity is filled with fat and marrow and is the relatively lucent portion in the X-ray, while the cortex of bone is seen as a white outline. The periosteum covers bone and is not seen in the X-ray. Some long bones, for example, femur, have a nonarticulating apophysis at the end of a protrusion of bone (greater trochanter). It is like an epiphysis, grows and fuses with the shaft, but does not contribute to linear growth of the bone.

ACCESSORY OSSICLES

These are accessory ossification centers. They are not always bilateral. Common accessory ossicles are the accessory navicular on the medial aspect of the foot near the navicular bone and os trigonum just behind the talus. Sesamoid bones are also accessory ossicles and are so named because they are shaped like sesame seeds. They are formed at the insertion of tendons and articulate with the adjacent bone. They help in reducing wear and tear of joints, tendons, and ligaments by reducing the tension on the tendons. The largest sesamoid bone in the body is the patella. Other sesamoids commonly seen in the knee are fabella (in the lateral head of the gastrocnemius muscle) and cyamella (in the head of the popliteus). In the foot, they are seen near the head of the first metatarsal.

SOME PECULIAR FEATURES IN THE GROWING SKELETON

It is essential to remember that bone X-ray of children, though largely similar to that of the adult, have some peculiarities arising out of its continuous growth. Many ossification centers are continuously appearing and fusing. These may appear fragmented as they ossify in a multicentric fashion and may thus simulate fractures. Likewise, certain epiphyses like that of the calcaneum appear fragmented and sclerotic and should not be mistaken for osteochondritis. The growth plate is a structure that should be preserved. Insults to the metaphysis-physis-epiphysis complex due to infection, trauma, or tumor are more damaging in the child as the growth plate is disturbed and linear growth of the child is altered. Salter Harris fractures are peculiar to children. These involve the growth plate. Since the child's capsular and ligamentous structures are five times stronger than the weakest part of the growth plate, the growth plate fractures first, and dislocations are less frequent. The zone of provisional calcification is the weakest part of the growth plate. Growing bones are "softer" and tend to bend before they fracture. The greenstick fracture consists of bending of bone, where there is a break on the convex surface while the concave surface is intact. In the torus fracture, there is buckling of one side of the cortex (Fig. 4.2).

In children, the periosteum is constantly growing so that it is loosely attached to the underlying cortex. Therefore, subperiosteal hematoma due to twisting injury or scurvy is more likely in children. For the same reason, the periosteum is easily lifted with accumulation of pus in osteomyelitis. The periosteum reacts by laying down new bone so that involucrum is exuberant in children.

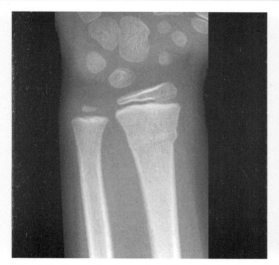

Fig. 4.2: Torus fracture—buckling of the lateral cortex of radius is seen.

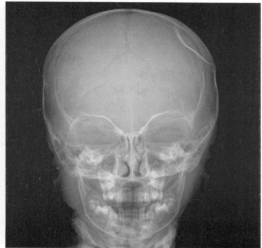

Fig. 4.3: Depressed fracture

The periosteum at the ends of bones is firmly adherent. So, twisting injuries here cause avulsion of a piece of bone from the metaphysis. Another difference between the adult and child is the ability to estimate bone maturation by studying the appearance and growth of epiphyses.

Depressed fracture (Fig. 4.3) of skull bones is common in children. Similarly, dural tear and growing fracture occur more readily in the child due to malleability of the growing skull and rapidly growing brain and skull causing close adherence of the dura to the bone. The arachnoid with the CSF bulges through the tear in the dura. This soft tissue interposition prevents dural and fracture healing. The pulsating pressure of the CSF erodes the edges of the fracture causing it to widen with time. An initial width of fracture more than 4 mm should alert the pediatrician to the possibility of a dural tear requiring follow-up. The growing fracture is seen as a wide gap with overlying soft tissue swelling representing the leptomeningeal cyst (Fig. 4.4).

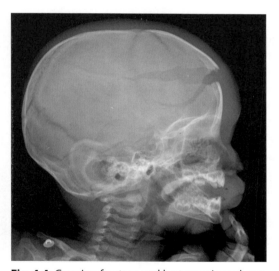

Fig. 4.4: Growing fracture and leptomeningeal cyst.

Estimation of Bone Age

There are two methods of evaluating precise bone age as reflected in specific X-rays. The Greulich and Pyle method uses the X-ray of the hand. It assesses the appearance of the various epiphyseal centers and changes in the shape of the bones as they grow. These have been standardized and documented and are available as an atlas. X-rays have to be matched with the standardized pictures. The other method is the Tanner and Whitehouse TW1 and TW2 (modified TW1) methods where numerical values have been assigned to growing bone patterns. This is considered to be more accurate but time consuming. The method that is being considered in this section is the oldest method that uses only the age of appearance of epiphyseal centers. This is what is used in forensic medicine and is generally familiar among students and clinicians. It can quickly separate those with growth disorders from the others. Further precise measurements can be done with either the Greulich and Pyle method or the TW method. These two methods are likely to be easier when computer-assisted techniques get more popular and available. Based on a large study in the Institute of Child Health and Hospital for Children, Chennai (Dr G Vijayalakshmi—unpublished data), the following pattern may be used. Depending on the chronological age of the child, specific X-rays are taken. Both hands with wrists, both knees anterior-posterior (AP) and lateral, and both elbows AP and lateral are taken. Knee X-rays can be excluded in children over 6 years of age. Elbows are taken if children are over 5 years of age. At birth, there are two centers in the hand—capitate and hamate. A preterm child may not have any centers in the hand. The knee X-ray will show the lower femur epiphysis that appears at the 36th week and the upper tibial epiphysis that appears at the 38th week. So, at birth, the X-ray of the knees is useful to evaluate hypothyroidism. The upper femur begins to ossify at about the 10th month and is seen as a well-defined round center by the age of 1 year. The carpal bones, with the exception of the pisiform, are very variable in their appearance. The pisiform appears by the age of 10 in girls and 11 in boys (Fig. 4.5). By 1 year 6 months, the distal radius is present. Though there is variability, it is definitely seen at 2 years. In contrast, the distal ulna is widely variable. All metacarpals appear by 2–3 years, but the second metacarpal is earlier by a few months. The base of the first metacarpal shows great constancy and can be used as a marker for 2 years 6 months.

In the elbow, the medial epicondyle appears by 7–8 years, the lateral epicondyle by 11 years. The olecranon is seen at about 10–10 years 6 months (Fig. 4.6). The radial head is definitely seen by 7 years and may appear at 6 years (Fig. 4.7).

There is a lack of indicators between the age groups of 3 years (seen in the hand) and 7 years (seen in the elbow). For this, the patella center can be used. A lateral X-ray of knees should be evaluated for the presence of the center for the patella. This shows great constancy and is seen by the age of four in both boys and girls. It should be remembered that epiphyseal centers in

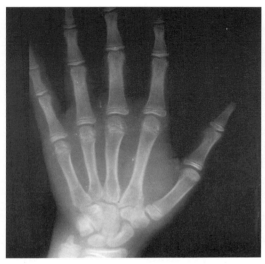

Fig. 4.5: Hand PA view. The pisiform has appeared.

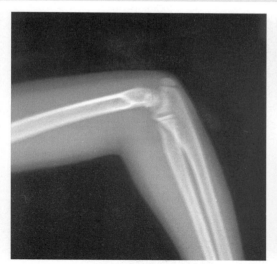

Fig. 4.6: Elbow lateral. Note the olecranon center.

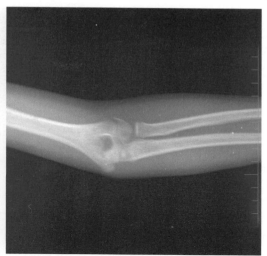

Fig. 4.7: The anteroposterior elbow shows the presence of radial head, medial, and lateral epicondyles.

general appear a little earlier in girls. But, the aforementioned centers do not show any remarkable difference between boys and girls (Fig. 4.8).

The triradiate cartilage fuses by 15 years (range 13–15 years) and the entire iliac crest appears by 16 years. In female children, it fuses soon after while in boys it may fuse only at 18 years (range 18–20 years). In general, ossification centers of long bones fuse by about 17 years.

Skeletal maturity is known to vary as much as 2 years on either side of chronological age in normal healthy children between ages 5 years and 14 years. So a discrepancy of more than 2 years is required to diagnose problems in maturation. After making an initial diagnosis using the aforementioned method, further accurate determination of bone age can be done when necessary by the other methods.

■ **CHROMOSOMAL DISEASES**

Turner's Syndrome

The genetic defect is a single X chromosome (45XO), partial deletion of X chromosome or

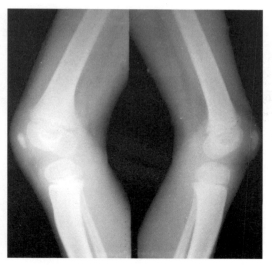

Fig. 4.8: Knees lateral for patella center.

mosaicism. The characteristic radiological sign is short fourth metacarpal giving rise to the metacarpal sign (Fig. 4.9). When a line drawn tangential to the heads of the fourth and fifth metacarpals is extended, it normally passes distal to the head of third

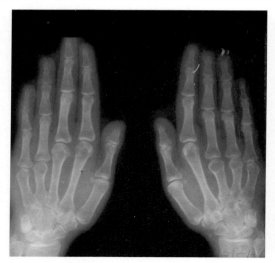

Fig. 4.9: Turner's syndrome. Note the short fourth and fifth metacarpals.

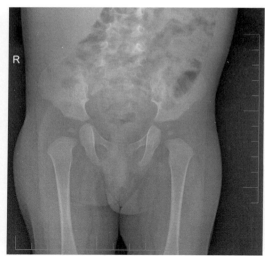

Fig. 4.10: Down's syndrome. Note the overhanging anterior superior iliac spine.

metacarpal. If it transects the head of the third metacarpal, the sign is positive as in Turner's syndrome. The fifth metacarpal can also be short. In older children, skeletal age is delayed.

■ NOONAN'S SYNDROME

This is the male phenotype of Turner's without chromosomal anomaly. There are short metacarpals and osteoporosis.

■ DOWN'S SYNDROME

The genetic defect is an extra 21 chromosome. The iliac wings are flared with horizontal acetabular roofs (Fig. 4.10). Sometimes there are 11 pairs of ribs. There may be mal-development of the dens with atlantoaxial instability. The skull is brachycephalic.

Trisomy 13, 18, and Cri Du Chat Syndrome

All these have microcephaly and microg-nathia. The pelvic bones are hypoplastic.

■ SKELETAL DYSPLASIAS

Skeletal dysplasias are a large group of disor-ders characterized by defective growth of bone and cartilage, which results in abnormality of the shape, size, and proportions of the skeleton. They are classified according to the skeletal abnormalities and more recently according to the underlying molecular genetic cause. The number of dysplasias is enormous and beyond the scope of this book. Some common dysplasias will be examined here. The first step is a clinical suspicion of a dysplasia. Short stature is a feature of most dysplasias. So, anthropometric measure-ments are necessary to decide whether proportionate or disproportionate shortening is present. Proportionate shortening is usually due to constitutional delay, familial short stature, endocrine disorders like growth hormone deficiency or hypothyroidism, as well as some congenital malformation syndromes. For this, skeletal maturation and bone age determination with X-ray is all that is required. When it is disproportionate shortening, radiological studies are called for. All the bones starting from the pelvis and axial skeleton to the limbs are studied. Essential X-rays are X-ray AP of the pelvis with both lower limbs, dorsolumbar spine AP and lateral, both hands PA and sometimes the skull. These X-rays help in coming to a conclusion in most cases. Further reference from specialty books can then be done.

Achondroplasia

Inheritance

❑ Autosomal dominant inheritance
❑ Common nonlethal dysplasia.

Radiological Features (Fig. 4.11)

Pelvis: The iliac wings are small and square. Acetabular roofs are horizontal. The sacrosciatic notches are narrow. Champagne glass appearance of pelvic brim.

Spine: The spinal canal is narrow. The interpedicular distance will taper downward

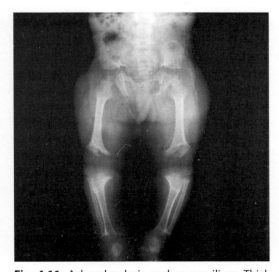

Fig. 4.11: Achondroplasia and square ilium. Thick short bones.

toward L5 or will remain parallel. This is the hallmark of achondroplasia. Normally the interpedicular distance widens from L1 to L5.

Long bones: Rhizomelic shortening, i.e. shortened proximal segments (humerus and femur). Bones are also thick. The upper femoral metaphysis is bulbous while the lower femoral metaphysis slants obliquely.

Hands: Metacarpals and phalanges are short and stubby.

Skull: The vault is large and base of skull is short.

Hypochondroplasia

Inheritance

❑ Autosomal dominant
❑ Genetically distinct from achondroplasia
❑ Clinically like mild form of achondroplasia, but skull and face are normal.

Radiological Features

Pelvis, spine, and bones similar to achondroplasia, but appears less severe. Skull is normal.

Thanatophoric Dysplasia

Inheritance

❑ Not certain
❑ The most common lethal dysplasia in newborns
❑ Severe short-limbed dwarfism.

Radiological Features

Pelvis: Pelvis as in achondroplasia (Fig. 4.12).

Spine: Flattened vertebral bodies. Narrow interpedicular distance like achondroplasia.

Long bones: Severe rhizomelic shortening. There is flaring at the metaphyses and bent shafts—telephone handle appearance.

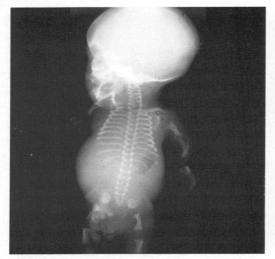

Fig. 4.12: Thanatophoric dysplasia. Flattened vertebrae and short bones with bent shafts.

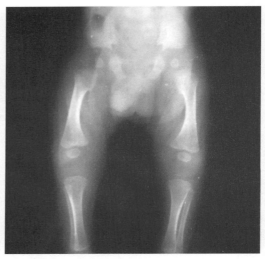

Fig. 4.13: Asphyxiating thoracic dysplasia—square ilium. Note the rounded upper femoral epiphysis.

Hands: Extremely shortened metacarpals and phalanges.

Skull: Skull base is short and vault is large with frontal bossing and cloverleaf appearance of the skull.

Asphyxiating Thoracic Dysplasia (Jeune's Disease)

Inheritance

❏ Autosomal recessive

Radiological Features

Pelvis: Iliac wings are squared as in achondroplasia (Fig. 4.13). Acetabular roofs show inferomedial projections at the sacrosciatic notches. Early appearance of the upper femoral epiphyses—a useful diagnostic feature.

Skull and spine: Normal.

Thorax: The ribs are extremely short causing respiratory embarrassment, the reason for the name (Fig. 4.14).

Long bones: Mild shortening. Hands: There may be polydactyly.

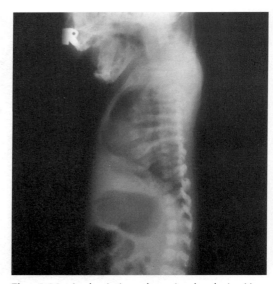

Fig. 4.14: Asphyxiating thoracic dysplasia. Very short ribs.

Chondroectodermal Dysplasia (Ellis-van Creveld Syndrome)

Inheritance

❏ Autosomal recessive

Radiological Features

Pelvis: Iliac wings are mildly squared. Acetabular roofs show inferomedial projections at the sacrosciatic notches as in asphyxiating thoracic dysplasia.

Skull and spine: Normal.

Thorax: Short and horizontal ribs giving a bell shape to the chest (Fig. 4.15).

Long bones: Mesomelic shortening. The proximal tibial epiphysis shows a medial slope (Fig. 4.16).

Hands: Short bones. Polydactyly, usually postaxial. Carpal fusions especially capitate and hamate. Delayed maturation of the carpal bones compared to the phalanges. In addition, dental abnormalities, hypoplastic nails, or sparse hair may be present.

Short Rib Polydactyly Syndromes

There are three distinct syndromes, but the common features are short ribs and preaxial polydactyly (Fig. 4.17). The additional features are as follows:

Type 1: Saldino-Noonan syndrome: Small iliac bones and short tubular bones.

Type 2: Majewski syndrome: Pelvis is normal, but femoral heads ossify early. Mesomelic shortening. Tibia is ovoid in shape (Fig. 4.18).

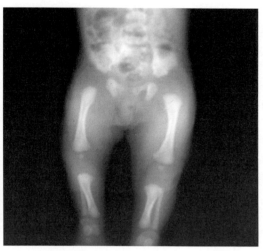

Fig. 4.16: Ellis-van Creveld syndrome—pelvis. Note the medially sloping metaphyses.

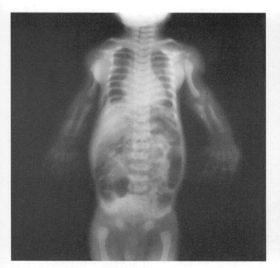

Fig. 4.15: Ellis-van Creveld syndrome. Bell-shaped chest and sloping metaphysis.

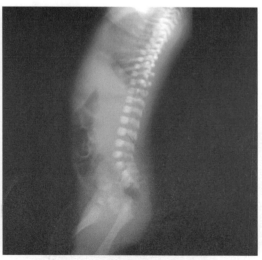

Fig. 4.17: Short rib polydactyly syndrome. Very short ribs.

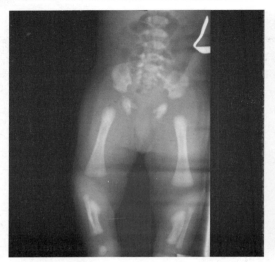

Fig. 4.18: Majewski type short rib polydactyly syndrome. Mesomelic shortening. Ovoid tibiae.

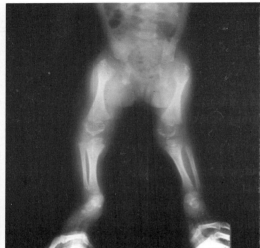

Fig. 4.19: Chondrodysplasia punctata. Stippled epiphysis.

Type 3: Verma-Naumoff syndrome: Short tubular bones, vertebral flattening.

Chondrodysplasia Punctata

Inheritance

There are three types:
1. Conradi-Hunermann—autosomal dominant
2. Rhizomelic form—autosomal dominant
3. X-linked form.

Radiological Features

Pelvis: Bones are normal. But multiple discrete punctate calcifications in the unossified epiphyses are seen (Fig. 4.19).

These may coalesce to form epiphysis or disappear by 3 years of age. Such stippling can be seen in other cartilaginous areas like trachea (Fig. 4.20).

Long bones: Rhizomelic shortening.

Hands: Stippling around the carpus.

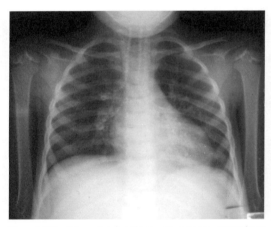

Fig. 4.20: Chondrodysplasia punctata. Stippling seen in the tracheal and bronchial cartilages.

Spine: Coronal cleft in vertebrae. Wedge-shaped vertebrae.

Skull: Normal

Metatropic Dysplasia

The name is due to the changing pattern of disease. At first dwarfism is due to short

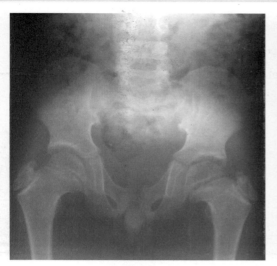

Fig. 4.21: Metatropic dysplasia—pelvis.

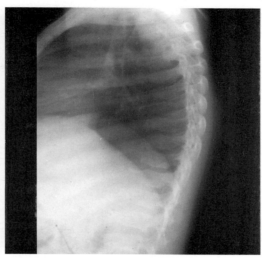

Fig. 4.22: Metatropic dysplasia—platyspondyly.

limbs. Later flattening of the vertebrae and kyphoscoliosis makes the trunk also short.

Radiological Features

Pelvis: The lower parts of the iliac bones are hypoplastic. Roof of acetabulum is horizontal and ischial and pubic bones are thick (Fig. 4.21).

Spine: Progressive platyspondyly. The anterior edges are more flattened or wedged (Fig. 4.22).

Long bones: Short with pronounced metaphyseal flaring.

Hands: Short with metaphyseal flaring (Fig. 4.23).

Thorax: Slightly narrow.

Skull: Normal.

Cleidocranial Dysplasia

Inheritance

☐ Mostly autosomal dominant, sometimes mutation

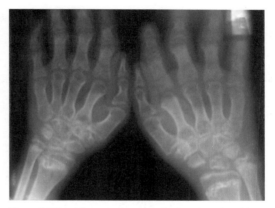

Fig. 4.23: Metatropic dysplasia—hands. Note widened metaphyseal ends.

Radiological Features

Pelvis: Symphyses apparently widened because the pubic bones show delayed ossification (Fig. 4.24).

Spine: Likewise, there is a persistence of the synchondroses between the neural arches and the vertebral bodies.

Thorax: Clavicles are hypoplastic or even absent. The ribs are a little short and scapulae are small (Fig. 4.25).

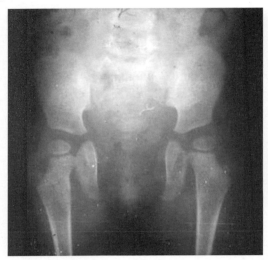

Fig. 4.24: Cleidocranial dysplasia. Pubic bones not ossified.

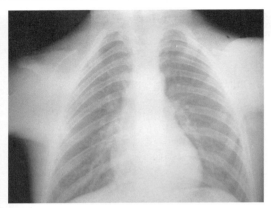

Fig. 4.25: Cleidocranial dysplasia. Absent clavicles.

Long bones: Normal.

Hands: The terminal phalanges are short. The second metacarpal is long. Accessory ossicles are present.

Skull: Delayed closure of anterior fontanelle. Many Wormian bones. Persistent metopic suture.

Metaphyseal Chondrodysplasia

This is a group of dysplasias characterized by abnormal metaphyses.

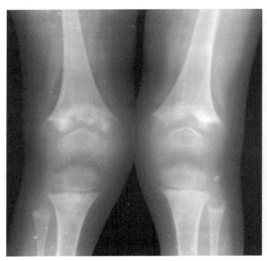

Fig. 4.26: Metaphyseal chondrodysplasia. Both femora and fibulae are involved. DD rickets in which all bones are involved.

Radiological Features

Pelvis: Normal.

Spine: Normal. In lateral view, the vertebral bodies may be ovoid.

Thorax: Normal.

Long bones: Flaring and irregularity of the metaphyses. The epiphyseal growth plate is apparently wide due to the dysplastic metaphyses (Fig. 4.26).

Hands: Likewise flaring and irregularity of metaphyses.

Skull: Normal. Schmidt type—aforementioned features, Jansen type—severe such features with skull base sclerosis, McKusick type (cartilage/hair hypoplasia)—additional feature is sparse hair. Pena type—longitudinal striations in the expanded metaphyses.

Shwachman syndrome—pancreatic lipomatoses and pancreatic insufficiency is the additional feature.

Metaphyseal Dysplasia

There is a lack of modeling of long bones causing expansion of the metaphysis and diaphysis giving the Erlenmeyer flask deformity. The short long bones can also be involved. This condition is an incidental finding. Pelvis and spine are normal.

Diaphyseal Dysplasia (Engelmann's Disease)

Pelvis is rarely involved. The long bones show sclerosis and thickening of the diaphyses, which narrows the medullary cavity. The epiphysis and metaphysis are not involved (Fig. 4.27). The short long bones also show similar changes. The spine is sclerotic.

Cerebrocostomandibular Syndrome

There is micrognathia just like Pierre Robin syndrome (Fig. 4.28). But, there are defects in the posterior parts of the ribs that cause respiratory distress (Fig. 4.29).

Ectodermal Dysplasia

This is an X-linked recessive condition characterized by hypohydrosis, hypotrichosis, and defective nails and complete or partial absence of teeth. The radiological finding is a lack of teeth seen in the lateral skull or mandible X-ray.

Disorders with Altered Density
Osteogenesis Imperfecta

This disorder consists of not only bone abnormality causing brittle bones, but also ligament laxity, dental abnormalities, and capillary fragility due to defect in Type 1

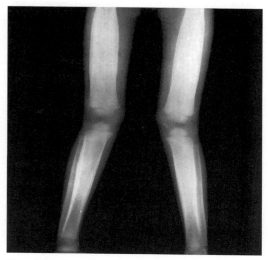

Fig. 4.27: Engelmann's disease. Thickened shafts of bone.

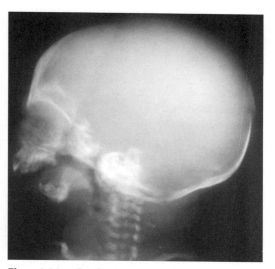

Fig. 4.28: Cerebrocostomandibular syndrome. Hypognathia.

collagen. It is classified into four types and further subtypes.

Type 1 is inherited as autosomal dominant. Bones are porotic. Sclerae are blue and there is deafness in adults. There is mild bone fragility. Fractures are not seen at birth, but

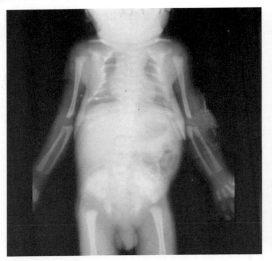

Fig. 4.29: Cerebrocostomandibular syndrome. Note the defects in the posterior part of the ribs.

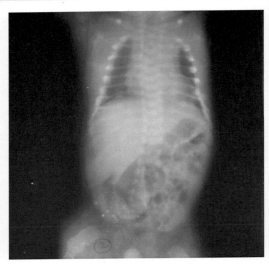

Fig. 4.30: Osteogenesis imperfecta. Thin gracile ribs.

develop later in preschool age up to puberty. Sometimes there are no fractures, but only some bowing.

Subtypes: Type 1A—teeth are normal. Bone fractures less. Type 1B—dentinogenesis imperfecta with more fragile bones.

Type 2—inheritance is due to new mutation which carries a risk of recurrence. It is a lethal type with severe osteoporosis and multiple fractures. The skull is large and poorly ossified, and sclera is deep blue.

Subtypes: Type 2A—the long bones are short and thick with numerous fractures. Ribs are broad with continuous beading due to fractures. Type 2B—long bones similar to Type 1, but ribs do not show beading. Type 2C–long bones are thin with fractures and ribs are thin with beading.

Type 3—inheritance is due to new dominant mutation. There are fractures at birth with progressive osteoporosis, bowing, and deformity. The features of Type 1 are more pronounced. In addition, there may be vertebral flattening. Dentinogenesis imperfecta is present.

Type 4—sclerae are usually normal. Bone fragility is mild and consequently fractures are less frequent.

Radiological Features

Pelvis: Shape is normal.

Spine: Vertebral compressions

Thorax: Ribs show beading and fractures or are very thin (Fig. 4.30).

Long bones: Fractures, which heal with plenty of callus. This and a lack of modeling make bones appear thick (Fig. 4.31). Bones can also appear thin and gracile. Hands: Also show thin bones, may show fractures.

Skull: Can be poorly ossified as in lethal Type 2. Basilar invagination in Type 4. Otherwise normal. Wormian bones may be seen.

Osteopetrosis

This is characterized by dense bones. The defect is in the osteoclast, so that bone resorption and therefore remodeling is affected.

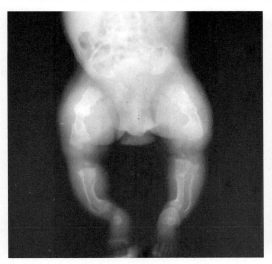

Fig. 4.31: Osteogenesis imperfecta. Porous bones. Multiple fractures with callus.

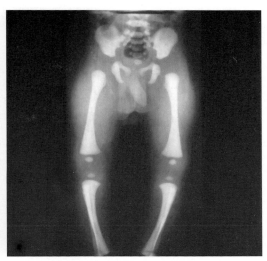

Fig. 4.32: Osteopetrosis—dense bones.

Bone encroaches on the marrow cavity, causing anemia and narrows neurovascular foramina causing cranial nerve palsies. A severe congenital recessive form presents with failure to thrive. Fractures may occur. The tarda dominant form may be discovered incidentally.

Radiological Features

Pelvis: Shape is normal but dense bones (Fig. 4.32). "Bone within Bone" appearance as old bone is not cleared by osteoclasts.

Spine: Sclerotic vertebrae. Central lucent horizontal stripe—Rugger Jersey spine.

Thorax: Ribs are thick and dense.

Long bones: Dense bones. Metaphysis may be club-shaped.

Hands: Bone within bone may be seen (Fig. 4.33).

Skull: Vault may be dense or skull base is dense.

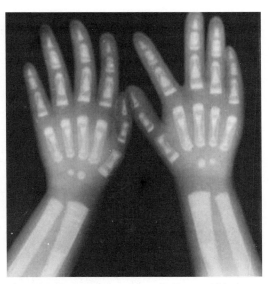

Fig. 4.33: Osteopetrosis—hands. Bone within bone appearance.

Pyknodysostosis

Inheritance

❐   Autosomal recessive

Radiological Features

Pelvis: Shape is normal. Dense bones (Fig. 4.34).

Spine: Sclerotic vertebrae.

Thorax: Clavicles may be thin.

Long bones: Sclerotic with tendency to fracture.

Hands: Terminal phalanges are small or absent (Fig. 4.35).

Skull: Dense vault and base. Persistent anterior fontanelle. The face appears small. The angle of the mandible is oblique (Fig. 4.36).

Melorheostosis

The characteristic radiological finding is linear sclerosis with cortical thickening along the diaphysis resembling dripping wax. The pelvis, ribs, and spine may be involved.

Dysostosis Multiplex Group

These include mucopolysaccharidosis, mucolipidosis, and storage diseases. Some have characteristic features. Once a suspicion of these is raised from X-ray, genetics and biochemistry will give the exact diagnosis.

Mucopolysaccharidoses [Hurler's Syndrome (1H)]

Radiological Features

Pelvis: Characteristic shape, signature of MPS—flaring of iliac wings and hypoplasia of lower part of iliac bones (Fig. 4.37).

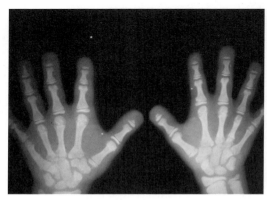

Fig. 4.35: Pyknodysostosis. Acro-osteolysis.

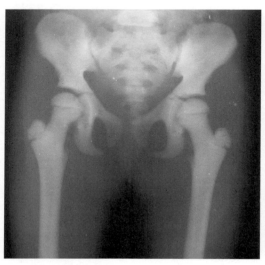

Fig. 4.34: Pyknodysostosis. Dense bones.

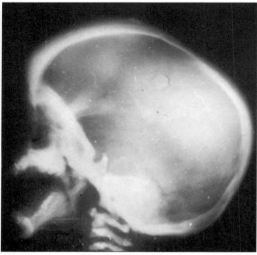

Fig. 4.36: Pyknodysostosis. Dense bones. Note the obtuse mandibular angle.

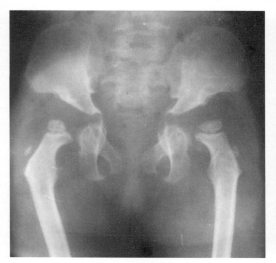

Fig. 4.37: Mucopolysaccharidoses—pelvis with hypoplastic lower ilium.

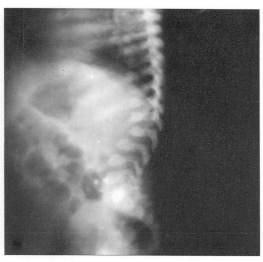

Fig. 4.38: Hurler's syndrome—spine. Inferior beaking of a few vertebrae.

Spine: Anterior beaking at the lower edge of the dorsolumbar vertebrae (Fig. 4.38). The dens may be hypoplastic, with atlantoaxial subluxation.

Thorax: Ribs are thick and spatulate, tapering posteriorly.

Long bones: Poor modeling.

Hands: Metacarpals are broad with tapered proximal ends and lack of the normal constriction in the middle (Fig. 4.39).

Morquio's Disease (MPSIV)

Radiological Features

Pelvis: Characteristic shape—flaring of iliac wings and hypoplasia of lower part of iliac bones. Acetabular fossae show irregularity.

Spine: Central anterior beaking of all the vertebrae, not just the dorsolumbar (Fig. 4.40). The dens may be hypoplastic with atlantoaxial subluxation.

Skull: Normal.

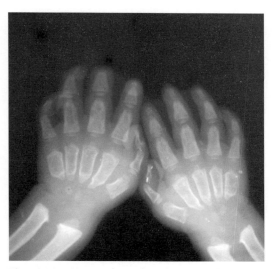

Fig. 4.39: Mucopolysaccharidosis—Hurler's syndrome of middle constriction.

Thorax: Ribs are thick and spatulate, tapering posteriorly.

Hands: Metacarpals are broad with tapered proximal ends and preservation of the normal constriction in the middle (Fig. 4.41).

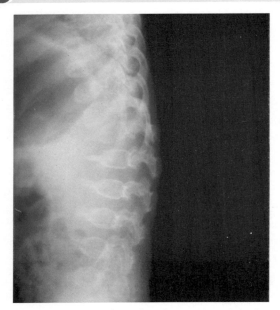

Fig. 4.40: Mucopolysaccharidoses. Morquio's disease. Flattened vertebrae with middle beaking.

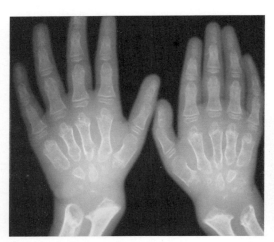

Fig. 4.41: Mucopolysaccharidoses. Morquio's disease tapering of metacarpals with maintenance of middle constriction.

All other mucopolysaccharidoses show the characteristic pelvis in varying severity. Other skeletal manifestations are absent or present in mild form.

Mucolipidosis

These are a group of disorders where enzyme defects lead to accumulation of metabolites and lysozymes. The clinical and radiological features are similar to mucopolysaccharidoses but more severe.

Radiological Features

Pelvis: Like MPS pelvis.

Long bones: Type 2 mucolipidosis or I-cell disease has a characteristic periosteal cloaking of the long bones present at infancy (Fig. 4.42). Mucolipidosis 1 is considered as the juvenile form of sialidosis. There is platyspondyly and metaphyseal irregularity. Then neonatal form presents with fetal hydrops. Mucolipidosis 3 or Pseudo-Hurler dysplasia presents with severe dysplastic changes of the bones. The clavicles are short, odontoid is hypoplastic, and tubular bones are short and thick. The metacarpals are short and middle wasting is preserved like

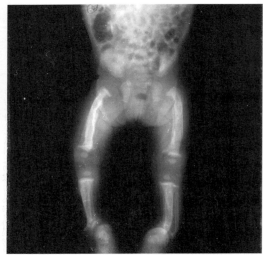

Fig. 4.42: Mucolipidosis type 2. Periosteal cloaking.

in Morquio's, but there is mental retardation like in Hurler's.

Certain Questions to Ask in Suspected Dysplasia

(1) Is it lethal? For homozygous achondroplasia, chondrodysplasia punctata (recessive form), congenital lethal hypophosphatasia, perinatal lethal type of osteogenesis imperfecta, thanatophoric dysplasia, and short rib polydactyly syndromes. (2) Shape of the pelvis—squared in achondroplasia, asphyxiating thoracic dystrophy, Ellis-van Creveld syndrome, MPS pelvis—mucopolysaccharidoses. (3) Shortening—rhizomelic shortening [short proximal segments (e.g. humerus and femur)], e.g. achondroplasia, hypochondroplasia, the rhizomelic type of chondrodysplasia punctata, the Jansen type of metaphyseal dysplasia, spondyloepiphyseal dysplasia congenita, thanatophoric dysplasia, and congenital short femur. Mesomelic shortening (short middle segments, e.g. radius, ulna, tibia, and fibula), mesomelic dysplasias, Ellis-van Creveld. (4) Short trunk indicates platyspondyly MPS and spondylometaphyseal and spondyloepiphyseal dysplasia. Long or narrow thorax—asphyxiating thoracic dysplasia and chondroectodermal dysplasia. (5) Large head—achondroplasia and thanatophoric dysplasia, cloverleaf skull—thanatophoric dysplasia. Multiple Wormian bones—cleidocranial dysplasia and osteogenesis imperfecta. (6) Hands-modeling defect—MPS, polydactyly—Ellis-van Creveld, hypoplastic nails—ectodermal dysplasia.

■ RICKETS

Bones are formed from cartilage. Most of the bones are ossified at birth except for the ends or the epiphyses, which remain cartilaginous. The secondary ossification center appears in the epiphysis and ossification proceeds radially around it. The part of cartilage in between the ossifying epiphysis and the metaphysis forms the growth plate, which is the lucent area seen in the X-ray between the radio-opaque epiphysis and metaphysis. It is the most active region where cartilage cells multiply, grow, calcify, and ossify in that order. The cartilage cells in the growth plate multiply and hypertrophy. The hypertrophied cartilage cells accumulate calcium. This is the zone of provisional calcification that is seen radiologically as the white line at the end of the metaphyses. In rachitic growth plates, calcium is reduced or absent and the provisional zone of calcification is lost. Normally osteoblasts along with capillary buds invade the area of calcified cartilage and lay down bone osteoid that later becomes mineralized. Calcium deposition in the bone depends on the supply of vitamin D. Vitamin D can be produced in the skin on exposure to sunlight. This is converted in the liver to 25-hydroxycholecalciferol and then in the kidney to the active 1-25, dihydroxycholecalciferol. The active form of vitamin D or D3 facilitates the absorption of calcium and deposition of calcium and phosphorus in growing bone. In rickets, while the osteoid is laid down normally, mineralization does not proceed due to the deficiency of vitamin D. The loss of the zone of provisional calcification and the loss of mineralization of bone osteoid widens the lucent area seen between the ossified epiphysis and metaphysis. This apparent widening of the growth plate is the hallmark of rickets. It is best seen at the knees, which is the most active growth plate (Fig. 4.43). The epiphysis of the knees is present at birth, so that the boundaries of the growth plate

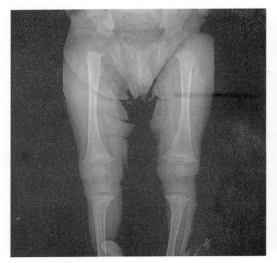

Fig. 4.43: Rickets. Note the increase in distance between epiphyses and metaphyses (widening of the physes).

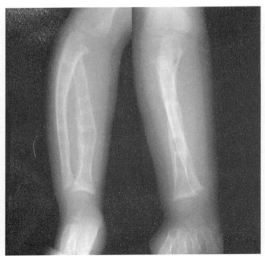

Fig. 4.45: Rickets with bowing of the radius at the site of healing fracture.

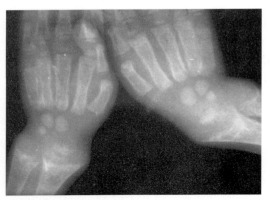

Fig. 4.44: Rickets. Note the increase in distance between epiphyses and metaphyses (widening of the physes).

are well defined radiologically. It is easy to appreciate the widening of the growth plate here. Where epiphyses are yet to be ossified, the nonossified gaps between contiguous bones at the joints appear wide (Fig. 4.44).

Cupping and splaying of the metaphyses is also seen. Cupping is due to the stress placed on the soft unmineralized bone matrix and is related to the degree of activity of the child, being more pronounced in the radius and ulna at the wrist in crawling babies. Fraying is due to irregular attempts to mineralize the cortex. There is thinning of the diaphyseal cortex and a general rarefaction of the bones (Fig. 4.45). Bending of bones especially lateral bowing of the tibiae can occur in advanced rickets.

Loosers zones seen in adults with vitamin D deficiency can be seen in children. They are small short radiolucent lines perpendicular to the surface of bones. They are stress fractures that have healed with callus lacking in calcium. They are usually seen in the neck of femur, pubic rami, and axillary edges of scapulae.

In the ribs cupping and splaying of the anterior ends occurs causing pressure microatelectasis of the underlying alveoli. This can be seen as white bands in both lungs along the anterior ends of the ribs—the radiological equivalent of the rickety rosary (Fig. 4.46). Frontal bossing is due to excess bone laid

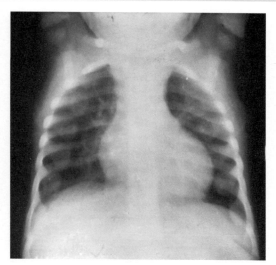

Fig. 4.46: Chest X-ray in rickets. Note the widened anterior ends of the ribs and the widened physes in the proximal humeri.

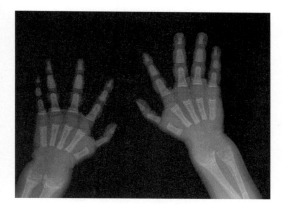

Fig. 4.47: Healing rickets. Reappearance of the zone of provisional calcification.

down without calcium. When rickets heals, it ossifies and is then seen in the X-ray.

With healing, the zone of provisional calcification reappears at the site it would normally appear if there were no interference with mineralization (Fig. 4.47). Then ossification progresses towards the shaft and the growth plate returns to a thin line. Deformities do not disappear completely.

On walking in children with severe rickets, the softened pelvic bones give rise to the triradiate pelvis that persists and is a cause for obstructed labor during childbirth. With better health standards and more awareness, dietary deficiency of Vitamin D is unusual. Other causes for rickets are malabsorption syndromes where there is failure of vitamin D absorption, impaired liver function which interferes with hydroxylation of the prohormone and long-term phenobarbitone therapy.

Vitamin D-dependent rickets: These are inherited disorders that present with rickets. In the Type 1 disorder there is a failure of hydroxylation in the kidney to the active 1,25-dihydroxy cholecalciferol. These children respond to doses of D3, but children with Type 2 do not. In Type 2 the level of 1,25-dihydroxy cholecalciferol is normal indicating end-organ resistance.

Vitamin D-resistant rickets: This is due to a group of genetic disorders causing renal tubular defects with impairment of phosphate reabsorption. The most common is the X-linked hypophosphatemic rickets. Phosphate supplements are required along with large doses of vitamin D. These children are short with features of rickets.

Oncogenic rickets: This is vitamin D-resistant rickets due to certain soft tissue tumors, such as nonossifying fibroma, osteoblastoma, giant cell tumors, hemangiomas, and hemangiopericytoma sand fibrous dysplasia. Following excision of the tumor, rickets regresses, and reappears with recurrence of the tumor.

Hypophosphatasia

It is a rare inborn error of metabolism characterized by low concentration of alkaline phosphatase isomer also called tissue nonspecific

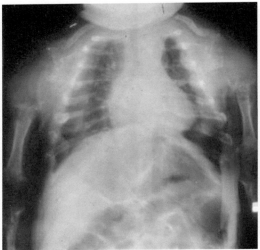

Fig. 4.48: Hypophosphatasia. Note the deep box like cupping. Here it is especially appreciable in the ankle.

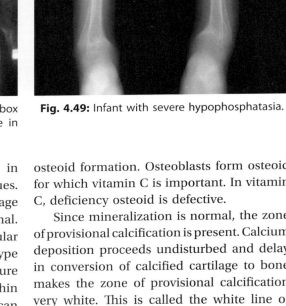

Fig. 4.49: Infant with severe hypophosphatasia.

alkaline phosphatase (TSALP) found in bone, liver, kidneys, and other tissues. There are four types depending on the age at presentation. The perinatal type is lethal. Skull bones are not ossified and tubular bones are extremely short. The infantile type presents in the first few months with failure to thrive and fractures. The ribs are thin and bones show poor ossification and can be confused with osteogenesis imperfecta (Fig. 4.48). The childhood type shows widening of the growth plate, with characteristic box-like defects in the metaphyses (Fig. 4.49). Other features are bent bones and fractures from trivial trauma. The adult type presents at middle age and they suffer from repeated stress fractures.

Scurvy

Scurvy is now seen only rarely, in neglected and mentally retarded children. Rickets involves failure of mineralization while osteoid formation is normal. Scurvy is a disorder of osteoid formation. Osteoblasts form osteoid for which vitamin C is important. In vitamin C, deficiency osteoid is defective.

Since mineralization is normal, the zone of provisional calcification is present. Calcium deposition proceeds undisturbed and delay in conversion of calcified cartilage to bone makes the zone of provisional calcification very white. This is called the white line of Frankel. The same reason holds good for the white line surrounding the epiphyses, called the Wimberger's sign, where growth of cartilage and bone formation takes place in a radial fashion. On the metaphyseal side of the white line is a lucent area of poorly formed bone matrix called the scorbutic zone or the zone of Trummerfeld. The scorbutic zone is seen first at the periphery of the metaphysis and presents as a lucent notch at the metaphyseal margin. Therefore, the white line of provisional calcification will appear to protrude beyond the edge of the metaphyses. This is the corner sign where subphyseal infractions and fractures can occur. These fractures heal with the formation of lateral spurs between the provisional zone of calcification and the shaft—the so called Pelken's spur (Fig. 4.50).

Preexisting bone undergoes resorption at a normal rate, but since new bone is not formed simultaneously, the bones become brittle. Small fractures occur, usually subphyseally. These fractures can cause subperiosteal hemorrhages lifting the periosteum away from the bone. Bleeds can be very large because vitamin C is essential for collagen formation and capillary endothelial stability. Hemorrhages can also be spontaneous as in the gums and skin.

Hypervitaminosis

These are rare. Hypervitaminosis A is possible because of common use of retinoids by dermatologists. It causes cortical thickening especially of the ulna and metatarsals. Hypervitaminosis D is possible during treatment of resistant rickets where large doses are given. It can cause cortical thickening, metastatic calcification, and nephrocalcinosis.

Heavy Metal Poisoning

Ingestion of lead is seen in children playing in scrap yards with dismantled used batteries. The characteristic feature in lead poisoning is the appearance of dense white transverse metaphyseal bands (Fig. 4.51). These are seen at all the sites of active bone growth—long bones, in the iliac crest, costochondral junctions, and inferior scapular edge. The anterior edges of the ribs and the manubrium are not usually seen very well in the chest X-ray, but in lead toxicity, they stand out prominently (Fig. 4.52). As the child grows and is removed from the lead source, the white band moves shaft wards and is seen separate from the zone of provisional calcification. In time, the white bands can disappear.

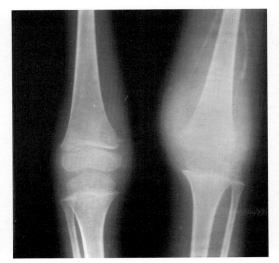

Fig. 4.50: Scurvy. Note the large periosteal hemorrhage lifting the periosteum on the left. Pelken's spur is seen in the lower right femur medially

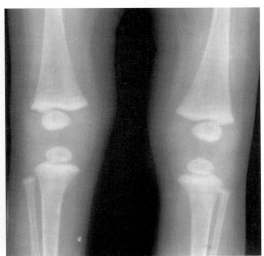

Fig. 4.51: Heavy metal poisoning. Note thick white metaphyseal bands.

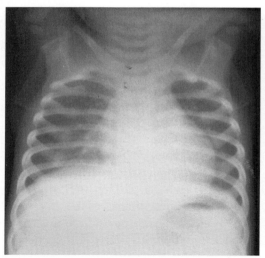

Fig. 4.52: Heavy metal poisoning. Note prominently white anterior ends of ribs and white lower border of scapula.

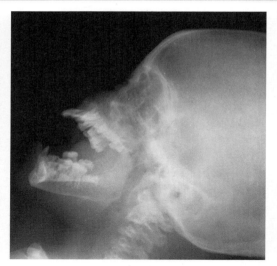

Fig. 4.53: Renal rickets. Subperiosteal resorption and loss of lamina dura (white line around roots of teeth are not seen).

Fluorosis

Fluorosis is a problem in many states where ground water is heavily contaminated with fluorides. Stiff and painful joints occur much before detectable radiologic signs. Fluoride is a cumulative poison causing increased bone turnover and defective collagen synthesis. The X-ray features are a combination of osteosclerosis of the axial skeleton, osteoporosis of the distal bones, and ossification of interosseous ligaments.

Renal Osteodystrophy

This develops when chronic renal disease causes failure of conversion of 25-hydroxy vitamin D to the active form. Phosphate excretion is also affected. The rising phosphate and low calcium due to reduced vitamin D3 causes a rise in parathormone excretion by the parathyroid gland. Parathormone mobilizes bone by resorption in an attempt to maintain calcium levels in the blood (Fig. 4.53). The radiological features are a combination of rickets and hyperparathyroidism. There is an apparent widening of the growth plates because of lack of calcification of osteoid. There are subperiosteal erosions in the middle phalanges of the index and middle fingers due to increased parathormone. The bones in renal rickets have a chalky white appearance due to excess of partly calcified osteoid. The radiological hallmark of renal rickets in children is the picture of rickets along with a delay in skeletal maturation.

Wilson's Disease

This is an autosomal recessive disorder of copper metabolism where there is impairment of the capacity of the liver to metabolize copper and excrete it in the bile. Renal copper levels are high and copper gets deposited in the central nervous system, liver, kidneys, and cornea. Renal copper deposition causes renal tubular damage, renal tubular acidosis, and as a consequence of this rickets develops.

BONE IN ENDOCRINE DISEASE
HYPOTHYROIDISM

The lower femoral epiphysis appears at 36th week and the upper tibial epiphysis appears at the 38th week. Consequently, at birth the term neonate shows the lower femoral and upper tibial epiphyses in an X-ray of the knees. In hypothyroidism, there is a delay in the appearance of epiphyses (Fig. 4.54) and eventually when it occurs, it ossifies from multiple centers. The epiphyses will appear flattened and fragmented (Fig. 4.55). This is best seen in the pelvis and is called epiphyseal dysgenesis. The acetabulum may also show mild irregularity. If untreated, epiphyseal fusion is delayed. The sella is enlarged due to hypertrophy of the pituitary gland for increased thyrotropin secretion in response to low thyroid hormone. Dental development is also delayed. The spine shows dorsolumbar kyphosis and mild flattening due to underdevelopment of the anterior aspects of the upper lumbar vertebrae. After treatment bone, maturation should be monitored.

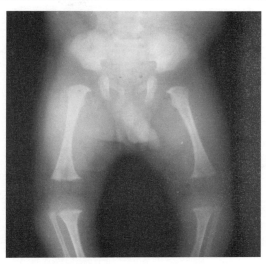

Fig. 4.54: Hypothyroidism—small infant. Knee epiphyses are not seen.

Hyperthyroidism

Hyperthyroidism is associated with accelerated bone age and early epiphyseal fusion.

Hypoparathyroidism

Hypoparathyroidism in the neonate may be a component of DiGeorge syndrome, which comprises of absence of parathyroid and thymus glands with immunodeficiency or other branchial arch abnormalities. There are no skeletal changes in early life. The biochemical findings are hypokalemia and hyperphosphatemia, which respond to parathormone. Pseudohypoparathyroidism is a metabolic disorder where there is

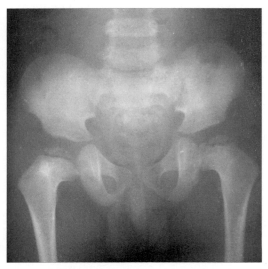

Fig. 4.55: Older child with hypothyroidism—delayed appearance of epiphyses and fragmentation.

hypokalemia and hyperphosphatemia, which do not respond very well to parathormone.

In pseudopseudohypoparathyroidism the biochemical findings are normal, but otherwise resemble pseudohypoparathyroidism.

Clinically both these conditions present with short stature, obesity, and mental retardation. There is intracranial calcification in basal ganglia and soft tissue calcification. The metatarsals and metacarpals are short particularly the fourth and fifth metacarpals.

Hyperparathyroidism

This is due to excess parathormone secretion. Primary hyperparathyroidism is due to tumor or hyperplasia of parathyroid glands. Secondary is when there is excess secretion of parathormone in response to chronic hypokalemia as in chronic renal disease. Tertiary hyperparathyroidism is due to autonomous parathyroid that occurs after a period of secondary hyperparathyroidism and prolonged stimulation of parathyroid glands. The features of this condition are the result of bone resorption by parathormone. These include general osteoporosis, subperiosteal erosions best seen in the radial aspect of the middle phalanges of the second and third fingers and medial aspect of the proximal tibial metaphyses. Erosions are also seen at the medial aspect of the clavicles, ribs, scapulae, and ischial tuberosities. Localized resorption gives rise to the pepper pot appearance in the vault of the skull. Brown tumors are again localized resorptions where the reparative process leads to accumulation of excess fibrous and vascular tissue. Osteoporosis can cause flattening of vertebrae. Excess circulating calcium can be deposited in the kidneys, walls of arteries, and in the brain.

Hypopituitarism

Dwarfing is proportionate. Bone age is retarded.

Hyperpituitarism

There is acceleration of growth and gigantism due to increased growth hormone. Skeletal maturation and epiphyseal fusion are sometimes delayed. Computerized tomography (CT) evaluation is to be done to study the sella and exclude pituitary tumor.

Adrenogenital Syndrome

There is accelerated skeletal maturation and premature fusion of epiphyses leading to short stature.

Cushing's Syndrome

Changes are due to adrenal tumor or steroid therapy. Generalized osteoporosis can cause fractures. There is excess fat deposition. Avascular necrosis (AVN) may occur, most often in the upper femoral epiphysis.

■ INFECTIONS OF BONES AND JOINTS

Infection of bone or osteomyelitis is caused by organisms that reach bone either directly due to trauma or more commonly hematogenous spread. The morbidity associated with the disease makes an early diagnosis very important.

Pathogenesis: The nutrient artery enters the shaft of the long bone through the nutrient foramina. Then it divides into two in the medullary cavity, the ascending and the descending branches. These further divide and then anastomose with the metaphyseal arteries. The metaphyseal arteries are perforating branches from nearby systemic vessels. Epiphyseal arteries are also perforating branches from periarticular vascular arcades. In the infant when the epiphysis is cartilaginous, the metaphyseal arteries pass freely into the epiphysis. Blood borne bacteria can come up to the articular surface and thus can gain access to the joint space. With progressive ossification of the epiphysis, metaphyseal vessels do not pass through the growth plate, but loop back to enter sinuses with sluggish blood flow which then drain into veins. A combination of high vascularity, hairpin-like looping of blood vessels and sluggish flow in the sinuses makes infection typically metaphyseal in this age (between 1 year and 16 years). Infection of the joint cannot occur by contiguous spread from here as the growth plate acts as a barrier. Joint infection in this age is by hematogenous spread or if the metaphysis happens to be intracapsular, as in the upper femur, distal fibula, and radial neck. As the child grows, the growth plate disappears as the epiphysis fuses with the metaphysis. Now continuity of epiphysis and metaphysis are reestablished and blood vessels also reanastomose. In adult life, infection of the joint again occurs directly from subarticular bone.

Acute Osteomyelitis

The initial radiographs do not show any abnormality. About 3 days after infection there is soft tissue swelling, which progresses in intensity in the next 3 days. The plane involved is the muscle plane without any subcutaneous edema. This is called the muscle sign (Fig. 4.56). In order to appreciate the soft tissue changes it is essential to X-ray the normal, as well as the abnormal side. The subcutaneous fat and the deeper muscle are well delineated in the radiograph. The muscle plane swelling has certain characteristics. It is circumferential which means it is seen on both sides of the bone in the X-ray. It is also seen along the entire length of the affected bone. At this stage, when the bone is drilled, pus is obtained as the suppurative

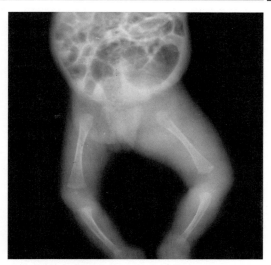

Fig. 4.56: Acute osteomyelitis—full circumferential swelling, along the entire length of bone (the muscle sign).

phase is well established. Although bone destruction is present, it is not seen in the X-ray. Treatment at this stage prevents massive bone destruction. The full-blown bone destruction and periosteal new bone formation is not seen until 10 days. It should be remembered that the amount of bone destruction seen in the X-ray is much less than what has actually occurred. These early radiographic signs of acute osteomyelitis are of great assistance in the early diagnosis of osteomyelitis and prevention of morbidity associated with chronic osteomyelitis.

Chronic Osteomyelitis

If pus is not drained from the bone, it accumulates in the medullary cavity. Bone is a rigid tissue and pus accumulating under great pressure breaks out through a hole in the bone and collects under the periosteum. Chronic osteomyelitis is irrevocably established at this

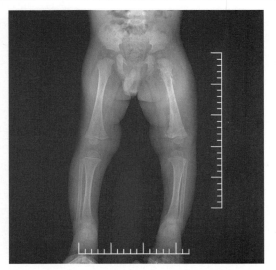

Fig. 4.57: Chronic osteomyelitis—there is destruction with periosteal thickening in left femur.

point. Bacterial organisms cause cell death and also cause infective thrombosis of the end-arteries of the metaphysis. Pus stripping the periosteum (Fig. 4.57) away from the bone also deprives the bone of supply from the periosteal arteries. These factors cause dead bone, which is called sequestrum. The stripped periosteum responds by producing new bone. This is the involucrum, which is prominent in children as the periosteum is not as adherent to the bone as in adults. Later this can become so extensive that it can form another shaft around the dying bone. As disease progresses, large areas of bone and sometimes the whole shaft can die and form large sequestra, floating in pus and surrounded by involucrum. The pus periodically discharges through openings in the involucrum called cloacae and through sinuses in the soft tissue to the skin. Radiological diagnosis is obvious at this point, but of little therapeutic use. Bony sequestrum is devitalized bone that has been separated from the surrounding

bone during the process of necrosis. The term "button sequestrum" has been used in calvarial lesions. Radiologically it appears as an area of calcification surrounded by a lucent ring. The dense area of calcification is because of the absence of blood supply that prevents any demineralization. The surrounding normal bone has retained its blood supply that enables demineralization. Some primary bone tumors produce a matrix that may mineralize and sometimes simulate a bone sequestrum. These include osteoid tumors like osteoid osteoma and osteoblastoma, cartilaginous tumors like chondroma and chondroblastoma; however, the associated clinical and other radiological findings enable a correct diagnosis.

Sclerosing Osteitis of Garre

This is a type of chronic osteomyelitis seen in children and young adults where there is a profuse osteoblastic response. The central medullary canal becomes dense, corticomedullary differentiation is lost, and there is exuberant periosteal new bone formation. There is no pus collection. Important differential diagnoses are osteosarcoma when in long bones and Ewing's tumor when in flat bones.

Brodie's Abscess

It is a type of subacute osteomyelitis where the patient's immunity balances the virulence of the organism. So the central lucent area of inflammatory necrosis is surrounded by a prominent zone of reactive sclerosis. The central area contains pus, which may be sterile. Lower limb bones are commonly affected especially the tibia. Brodie's abscess can cross the growth plate. Differential diagnoses include osteoid osteoma and osteoblastoma or chondroblastoma.

Septic Arthritis

Joints can be infected hematogenously or from the adjacent bone. Timely diagnosis is essential to prevent morbidity. Radiologically, there is soft tissue swelling around the joint with loss of fat planes. There is increased density of the soft tissue (Fig. 4.58). At this stage, the diagnosis has to be made and the joint should be aspirated and relieved of pus. Accumulation of pus causes dislocation of the joint as is seen in the case of the hip joint where the acetabulum is not yet fully developed and the femoral head is displaced superiorly and laterally (Fig. 4.59). Epiphyses may be completely destroyed never to reappear. Growth plate can be destroyed and growth is affected.

Tuberculous Osteomyelitis

Tuberculous osteomyelitis involves mainly the thoracic and lumbar vertebrae, followed by knee and hip. There is a focus of lytic destruction in the metaphysis of long bones. Sequestra may be present. There is a very thin zone of reactive sclerosis around the lesion. Sclerosis that is seen in pyogenic osteomyelitis is conspicuously absent and this is a useful differentiating feature. The infection can traverse the growth plate and spread into the epiphysis contrary to pyogenic osteomyelitis.

In short, long bone tuberculous infection results in a peculiar appearance of a widened bone with a lucent center. This is called spina ventosa (Fig. 4.60). The infection begins in the middle of the shaft because the nutrient artery breaks into a plexus of vessels immediately on reaching the medullary cavity, unlike in the long bones where the artery divides into two branches, which ascend or descend to the metaphyseal ends of bones. This picture is not seen in adults as the nutrient artery is replaced by periosteal vessels along the length of the bone. Multiple bones may be affected and it is more common in children below 5 years of age.

Tuberculosis of Joints

At first, there is synovitis with joint swelling. Inflammation results in hyperemia that

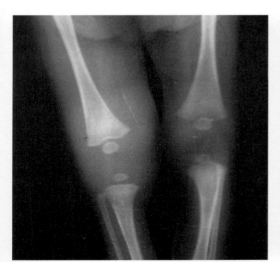

Fig. 4.58: Septic arthritis of the knee. Note the soft tissue swelling around the knee joint.

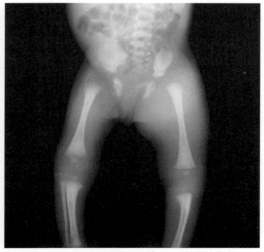

Fig. 4.59: Septic arthritis left hip with hip dislocation and acute osteomyelitis of left femur.

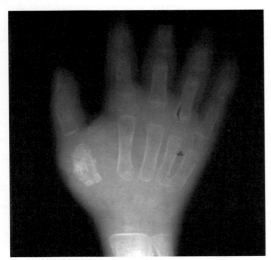

Fig. 4.60: An expanded first metacarpal with destruction—spina ventosa.

may cause an overgrowth of the epiphysis. This is also seen in juvenile arthritis, which is a differential diagnosis. Cartilage undergoes necrosis-causing narrowing of the joint space. The epiphysis is eroded and destroyed. Pus escapes from the joint space and forms periarticular cold abscesses. Synovial tuberculosis may occur without obvious bone involvement in the X-ray. The diagnosis is made by synovial biopsy.

Spinal Tuberculosis

The spine is the most common site involved in skeletal tuberculosis. The bacillus spreads by the hematogenous route and lodges in the cancellous bone of the vertebral body. Sometimes the starting focus of infection is in the anterior body below the anterior longitudinal ligament. Occasionally the posterior arch or transverse process can be involved. With progressive infective destruction, the vertebral body loses its mechanical strength and collapses, causing local kyphosis. Anterior collapse results in anterior wedging, while collapse of the posterior body is seen as

close approximation of the ribs. The posterior arch and intervertebral joints are preserved. Kyphosis is most marked in the thoracic area, because of exaggeration of the normal dorsal curvature. In the lumbar region, it is opposed by normal lumbar lordosis. Collapse is minimal in the cervical spine, because body weight is normally transmitted through the articular processes.

From the initial focus just beneath the endplate, infection extends to the end plate and through the intervertebral discs, causing contiguous spread to multiple vertebrae. Narrowing of the disk space is a hallmark of tuberculous infection of vertebrae (Fig. 4.61). The caseous material may breakthrough and cause large paraspinal abscesses. These gravitate along fascial planes to present at a site far from the infected site. In the lumbar region, the abscess gravitates along the psoas fascial sheath and usually points into the groin just below the inguinal ligament. In the thoracic region, it is seen in the X-ray as a fusiform, radiopaque shadow at or just below the level of the involved vertebra (Fig. 4.62). Thoracic

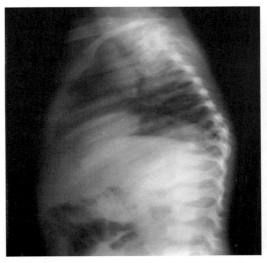

Fig. 4.61: Caries spine—reduced disk space between D9 and D10 and a localized gibbus.

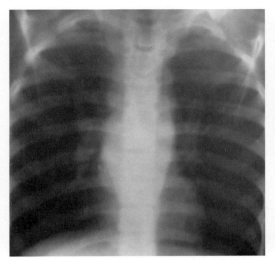

Fig. 4.62: Caries spine—paraspinal soft tissue shadow—cold abscess.

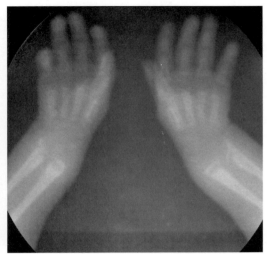

Fig. 4.63: Horizontal lucent bands in the metaphysis—metaphysitis of syphilis.

abscess may reach the anterior chest wall in the parasternal area by tracking via the intercostal vessels. Progressive destruction, fibrosis, and fusion of contiguous vertebrae cause progressive kyphosis. Vertebral body collapse and narrowing of disk space are features of spinal tuberculosis.

Syphilis

Syphilis is rare in present times, but not unheard of. The lesions of congenital syphilis consist of metaphysitis, diaphysitis, and periostitis. The epiphysis is not involved.

Metaphysitis may consist of a transverse lucent band (Fig. 4.63) or vertical lucencies like rubella. Focal bone destruction is seen in the metaphyses around the knee or shoulder. The characteristic punched out defect of the medial metaphysis seen in the upper tibia is called the Wimberger sign (Fig. 4.64). Periostitis consists of lamellar periosteal reactions and new bone formation that is seen in most bones.

Diaphysitis is not usually obvious radiologically, but lytic lesions can occur in the

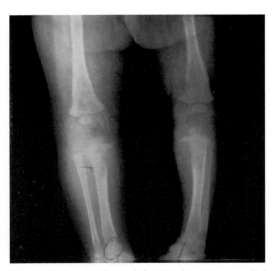

Fig. 4.64: Punched out defect in the upper medial tibia—Wimberger sign.

medulla or destruction can extend from the metaphysis. A picture similar to tuberculous spina ventosa may occur, but bone proliferation dominates over destruction. Since this is a systemic disease, there is widespread involvement of bones. Lesions are bilateral and symmetric. With or without treatment, lesions regress. These features of early disease are seen in the neonate, but can be seen up to 2 years of age. Late lesions consist of gummata that are seen as lucent defects in the bone and a severe lamellar periostitis with new bone formation. Painless effusions in the knee are called Clutton's joints.

Rubella

Some children with congenital rubella syndrome develop a few changes that are also associated with other viral infections including cytomegalovirus. These consist of metaphyseal lucencies with alternating vertical bands of lucency and density extending into the diaphysis—the celery stalk appearance.

Pyomyositis

Tropical pyomyositis is a bacterial infection of the muscles. Lower limbs are usually involved. Age group affected is 10–30 years. Skeletal muscle is usually quite resistant to infection, but a combination of prior injury and transient bacteremia in the tropics is associated with pyomyositis. Initially, there is fever and muscle pain and no pus. Later pus collects in the muscle plane and should be aspirated. A high index of suspicion is necessary, as it mimics acute osteomyelitis.

■ NEOPLASIA OF BONES

Bone Tumors

Malignant bone tumors are rare in children. The common ones are benign.

Benign Bone Tumors

The simple bone cyst is seen as a lucent defect in the metaphysis of long bone near

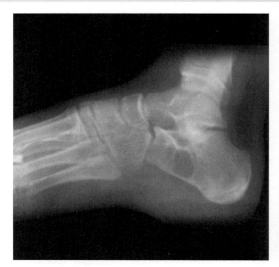

Fig. 4.65: Bone cyst in the calcaneum.

the growth plate. It is most often found in the humerus, femur, or tibia. Another common location is the calcaneus (Fig. 4.65). It has a well-defined sclerotic margin. Thinning of the cortex can cause a pathological fracture. A fracture fragment within the cyst can give the falling leaf sign. The aneurysmal bone cyst is an expansile lytic lesion seen in long bones and posterior spinal elements. Before epiphyseal closure, it is seen in the metaphysis (Fig. 4.66).

Once the epiphyseal plate closes it can involve the epiphysis also. There is a thin sclerotic rim that may be seen well only in CT especially in spinal lesions. Pathological fractures are common. The fibrous cortical defect is a well-circumscribed, oval lucent lesion within the cortex at the end of a long bone, particularly the femur or tibia. The larger ones are called nonossifying fibromas (Fig. 4.67).

Osteochondroma

Osteochondroma (exostosis) is a protuberant cartilaginous growth arising from the

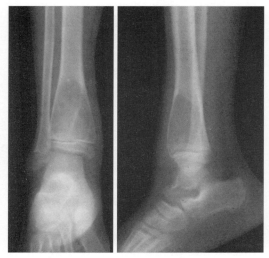

Fig. 4.66: Aneurysmal bone cyst in the tibia.

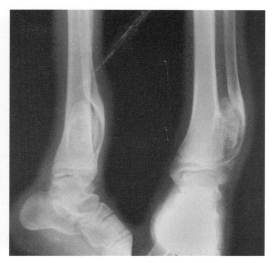

Fig. 4.68: Exostosis from the fibula.

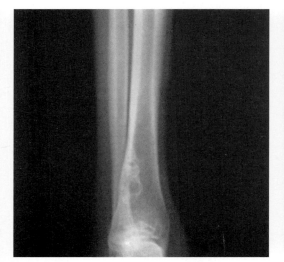

Fig. 4.67: Nonossifying fibroma in the cortex of the tibia.

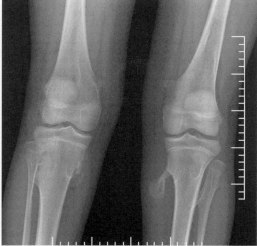

Fig. 4.69: Multiple exostoses.

meta-physis. It ossifies progressively and its cartilage cap tends to grow along with the child. The cortex can be traced in continuity with the cortex of the bone and the medullary cavity is also continuous with that of the parent bone (Fig. 4.68). They point away from the joint and commonly occur around the knee joints, hips, and shoulder. It can occur in flat bones also and can be multiple (Fig. 4.69).

Enchondroma

Enchondroma is a cartilaginous, cyst-like lesion often seen in the phalanges and rib.

They arise in the marrow, expand the bone, and may cause a secondary fracture. Multiple enchondromas, in a predominantly unilateral distribution constitutes Ollier's disease. When associated with multiple soft tissue angiomas, it is called Maffucci's syndrome, which carries with it an increased incidence of malignant transformation.

Osteoid Osteoma

The osteoid osteoma is a sclerotic lesion with a central lucent nidus. The lucent nidus consists of some osteoid, vascular, and fibrous tissue. It occurs in many places, involving the long bones and spine. The most common sites are tibia and femur (Fig. 4.70). The usual age of incidence is 5–25 years. It typically causes dull pain that is worse at night and is relieved by aspirin. Radiologically, it is seen as an oval or round lucency in the cortex of the shaft of the bone surrounded by an intense sclerotic region. The cortex is thickened. CT is very effective in showing the nidus, which has to be removed for relief of symptoms. When it occurs in the intramedullary region sclerosis is not marked as is seen in the neck of femur. Then the differential diagnosis includes Brodie's abscess and osteoblastoma. In the spine, it occurs more often in the posterior elements. An expanded sclerotic pedicle indicates osteoid osteoma.

Osteoblastoma

Osteoblastoma can be considered as a large osteoid osteoma. The osteoblastoma arises in the medulla. Common bones involved are posterior spinal elements, long bones, and jaw.

Osteofibrous Dysplasia

Osteofibrous dysplasia is a benign tumor involves tibia or fibula. There are multiple cyst-like lucent are as in the cortex of the shaft. It used to be considered as a type of fibrous dysplasia. It tends to recur on curettage, but regresses spontaneously if surgical removal is withheld.

Fibrous Dysplasia

Fibrous dysplasia appears as lucent defects with a hazy ground glass appearance within a sclerotic border. The affected part is soft and fractures easily. Sometimes it occurs as a dense sclerotic patch, commonly in the femoral neck, causing coxa vara. Monostotic fibrous dysplasia is seen commonly in the proximal femur, tibia, and ribs (Figs. 4.71 and 4.72). In the polyostotic type, many bones are involved. The skull may show thickening of the vault, base, or facial bones. The spine and thorax are rarely involved. Polyostotic fibrous dysplasia with sexual precocity and skin pigmentation is called McCune Albright syndrome. It has a slight female preponderance (Male:Female, 2:3).

Neurofibromatosis

There are two forms. Type 1 is the common peripheral form while type 2 is the central

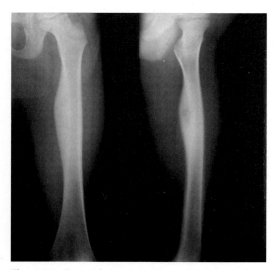

Fig. 4.70: Osteoid osteoma. Note the lucent nidus and surrounding intense sclerosis.

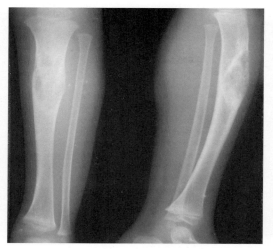

Fig. 4.71: Fibrous dysplasia.

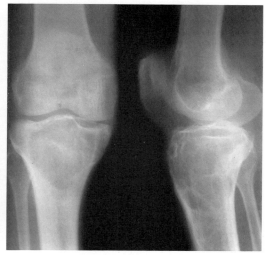

Fig. 4.73: Osteoclastoma of the tibia. Note the typical location and subchondral extension.

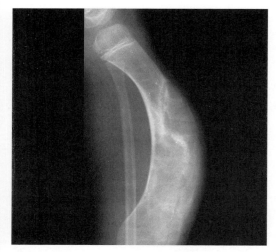

Fig. 4.72: Fibrous dysplasia involving the tibia.

form with central nervous system abnormalities like acoustic neuromas, gliomas, and meningiomas. Bowing and pseudoarthrosis is common in the tibia. Neurofibromatosis should be considered in any child with anterolateral bending of the tibia or both bones of the leg while posteromedial bending is due to intrauterine constricting bands. Intraosseous neurofibromas can also be seen as filling defects.

Giant Cell Tumor or Osteoclastoma

It is rare in childhood. It is seen as an eccentrically placed, expansile lytic lesion at the ends of long bones. It involves the epiphyses and extends up to the subchondral bone (Fig. 4.73). In childhood, it has a predilection for the scapula. Osteoclastomas may be quite aggressive, recur after curettage, and even metastasize to the lungs.

Malignant Bone Tumors

Osteosarcoma

This rare primary malignant bone tumor is seen usually in the 2nd and 3rd decades, and is more common in males. It occurs more around the knee, which are the regions of maximal growth. The characteristic radiological feature of this tumor is the formation of new bone. This new bone formation takes many appearances. It is seen as linear streaks perpendicular to the long bone—sunray appearance or multiple layers of periosteal reaction or raised periosteum with

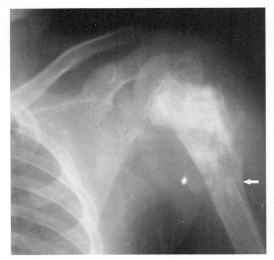

Fig. 4.74: Osteogenic sarcoma. Destruction of cortex and new bone formation. Note Codman's triangle (arrow).

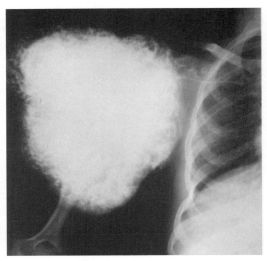

Fig. 4.75: Osteogenic sarcoma. Exuberant new bone formation.

Codman's triangle (Fig. 4.74). A number of variants of osteosarcoma exist, including conventional types (osteoblastic, chondroblastic, and fibroblastic), telangiectatic, multifocal, parosteal, and periosteal. The most common type is the conventional osteosarcoma (Fig. 4.75). The lesion starts in the medulla with irregular cortical destruction along with new bone formation (Fig. 4.76). Some osteosarcomas like the telangiectatic type are mainly lytic without new bone formation. Paraosteal juxtacortical osteosarcoma arises on the surface of the bone. Initially, it appears separate from the bone and should not be mistaken for myositis ossificans. Osteosarcomas metastasize to the lungs. These are round lesions that may calcify and cavitate. Cavitation can lead to pneumothorax.

Ewing's Tumor

This is the second most common tumor in pediatric age group. It is more common

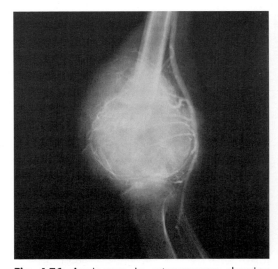

Fig. 4.76: Angiogram in osteosarcoma showing profuse neovascularity.

than osteogenic sarcoma in those under 10 years of age. It may occur in any bone, but the typical location in young children is the diaphysis of long bones. Other bones affected are vertebrae, ribs (Fig. 4.77), pelvis, and scapulae. The lesion starts in the medulla and the cortical destruction is permeative with ill-defined margins. New bone formation is also a feature of Ewing's sarcoma just as the osteosarcoma. This may be in the form of multilayered onion-peel periosteal reaction or bony spicules. There is a large soft tissue component.

Skeletal Metastasis

Metastatic neuroblastoma, retinoblastoma, and hepatoblastoma cause irregular lytic destructions with ill-defined edges.

Neuroblastoma secondaries commonly occur in the skull, long bone, spine, ribs, and pelvis. Retinoblastoma secondaries can be osteolytic and osteoblastic. Hodgkin's disease can also cause lytic secondaries in the spine and pelvis.

Leukemic bone deposits: These are seen as lytic transverse bands in the metaphysis (Fig. 4.78). Vertebral secondaries can cause compressions (Figs. 4.79 and 4.80).

The X-ray shows the location, size, and number of lesions. The characteristics of the lesion—whether benign or malignant—may also be inferred to a large extent. Only a biopsy can give the true diagnosis. Clear signs of a benign lesion include sharp demarcation between the lesion and the normal bone and sclerotic margin around the lesion. The characteristics most often associated with a malignancy include an accompanying soft tissue mass, periosteal reaction, an indistinct margin, and permeative destructive changes in the cortex.

■ MISCELLANEOUS

Avascular Necrosis

Avascular necrosis occurs when the blood supply to a part of the bone is cut off. There are many causes. A fracture of the femoral neck can lead to AVN of the femoral head. A fracture of the waist of the scaphoid leads to AVN of the distal part. These examples are

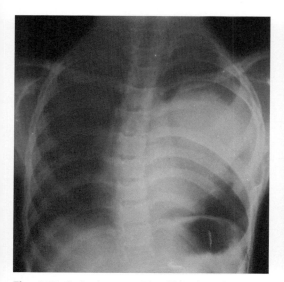

Fig. 4.77: Ewing's tumor. The fifth rib is destroyed and there is a large soft tissue shadow.

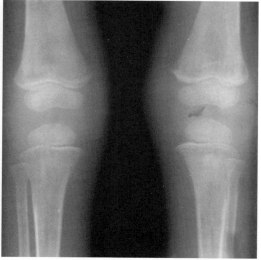

Fig. 4.78: Leukemic bone deposits. Lucent transverse metaphyseal bands.

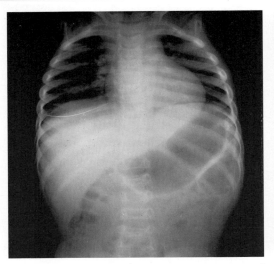

Fig. 4.79: Secondaries causing compression of multiple vertebrae (anteroposterior view).

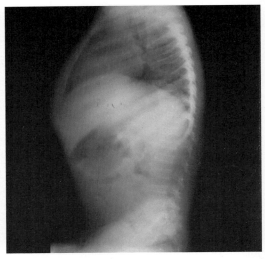

Fig. 4.80: Secondaries causing compression of multiple vertebrae (lateral view).

due to the course of the sole vascular supply without supply from alternate arteries. The lateral two-thirds of the femoral head is supplied by the lateral epiphyseal arteries, which are branches of the medial circumflex artery from the profunda femoris. They enter the head of the femur between the cartilaginous head and the cortical bone of the neck where they are likely to be interrupted in a fracture of neck of femur or with slipping of the capital epiphysis. The medial one-third is supplied from the artery of the ligamentum teres. There is anastomosis between these two arteries. In sickle cell disease, Gaucher's disease, hemoglobinopathies, and chronic steroid use there is arterial occlusion. In children when the head of the femur is undergoing development, most of it is cartilaginous. Unlike other connective tissue, cartilage does not contain blood vessels and is supplied by diffusion. The artery of the ligamentum teres does not penetrate the epiphysis of the femoral head until age 9–10 years. The medial circumflex comes up to the metaphysis, but does not cross the growth plate to supply the epiphysis. These reasons make the femoral head particularly vulnerable to AVN.

Osteochondroses

The osteochondroses are a group of disorders characterized by fragmentation and flattening of epiphyses. The pathology can involve long bones, round bones, sesamoids, an apophysis, or site of tendinous attachment. The cause is AVN following trauma though some are normal variants, e.g. Sever's disease. After a variable period, there is regeneration and recalcification.

Perthes Disease

This is AVN of the femoral head. The cause is not precisely known. The age of incidence is between 5 years and 10 years and there is a male preponderance of 4:1. It is bilateral in 10%. The changes in the femoral head can be followed in the anteroposterior plain X-ray of the pelvis, with care taken for genital shielding. Other views that can be taken are frog lateral view (45° abduction and external rotation), to view the superior aspect of the femur for fissure fractures. Initially, there is a widening of the joint space. The femoral head appears whiter. In the next phase, there is fragmentation of the femoral head so that it appears moth- eaten. During this phase, there is a return of blood supply. Healing then commences. The degree of lasting deformity depends on the amount of tissue that has undergone ischemia. This can be inferred from the length of the fissuring or by scintigraphy. In the bone scan, there will be reduced uptake in the blood pool phase. Magnetic resonance imaging (MRI) will also show the extent of AVN. If less than half the head is involved, the prognosis is good. If more is involved, the head shows pronounced collapse (Fig. 4.81). With healing, the head becomes increasingly sclerotic, followed by resorption of the sclerotic bone and reossification. The healed femoral head and neck become broad (coxa magna deformity), so that the lateral part of the head gets excluded from the acetabulum. This has to be surgically corrected to avoid lasting disability. The whole process of Perthes disease and healing can take months to years. Residual deformity leads to early osteoarthritic changes.

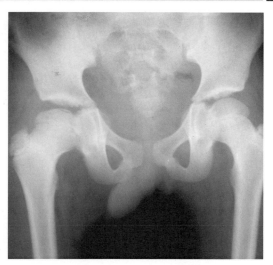

Fig. 4.81: Perthes disease. Reduction in height of epiphysis on right. Note the fissure in the epiphysis.

Kohler's Disease

There is a history of trauma. In this, the navicular bone is fragmented, flattened, and sclerotic. The navicular bone commonly shows irregular ossification and should not be confused with Kohler's disease. Comparison with the opposite side and the presence of pain are helpful.

Sever's Disease

This is a developmental variant, as the calcaneum is subject to weight-bearing stresses. It is therefore normally fragmented and sclerotic. A clinical diagnosis of Sever's disease can be made based on a painful heel.

Sinding Larsen Disease

This is AVN of the lower pole of the patella. There is a history of avulsion injury. There is fragmentation of the lower patella with soft tissue swelling and pain.

Osgood-Schlatter Disease

The involved bone is the tibial tubercle. The tibial tubercle normally shows fragmentation. So a diagnosis can be made on clinical grounds of pain and swelling.

Freiberg' Disease

The AVN involves the heads of the second and third metatarsals in older children. There is a history of trauma.

Panner's Disease

There is a history of trauma. The involved bone is the capitulum, which shows increased density, fragmentation, flattening, and sclerosis followed by healing. There is no residual deformity.

Thiemann's Disease

This is a familial condition affecting males more than females. The involved bones are the epiphyseal ossification centers of the phalanges, particularly of the middle fingers. The affected fingers are shortened.

Friedreich's Disease

The cause is not known. There is AVN of the medial end of the clavicle. Pain is a prominent symptom. There is some destruction of bone followed by healing.

Scheuermann's Disease

This condition consists of kyphosis and one or more anteriorly wedged vertebrae. The vertebrae involved are those between D3 and D12. The cause is not known, though it is grouped under osteochondroses. Pathologically, there are small fissures in the vertebral end-plate cartilage through which the nucleus pulposus herniates. The disk is therefore narrowed. Scoliosis may be present with kyphosis.

Blount's Disease

The parts of the bone involved are the medial metaphysis, growth plate, and epiphysis of the tibia. It usually occurs in infancy or in children less than 3 years when it is called infantile type. AVN has not been demonstrated. Early walking even as developmental bowing is taking place causes unusual stress and disordered growth of the medial tibia at the knee. Juvenile Blount's disease is associated with obesity. On radiographic examination, there is beaking of the medial

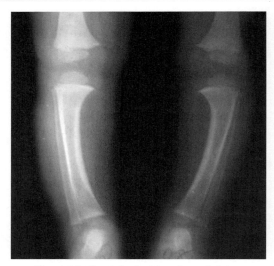

Fig. 4.82: Physiological bowing of tibiae.

tibial metaphysis with a sharp angle where the beak meets the shaft. There is lateral bowing of the tibia or genu varus, which is different from physiological bowing (Fig. 4.82).

Physiological genu varum consists of external rotation of the thigh with internal tibial torsion. The peak of the bowing is in the mid-shaft and the deformity resolves spontaneously by the age of 2 years. In Blount's disease, the peak of bowing is more proximal and there may be progressive deformity (Fig. 4.83).

Child Abuse/Nonaccidental Injury

The important musculoskeletal feature of nonaccidental injury is the presence of multiple fractures in various stages of healing. The classical fractures are metaphyseal fractures, which appear as chip fractures or "corner" fractures. The severe type is the bucket handle fracture where a rim of metaphysis is separated. Shearing forces from shaking and twisting tear through the metaphyses adjacent to the growth plate, which is the most recently ossified and, therefore, the

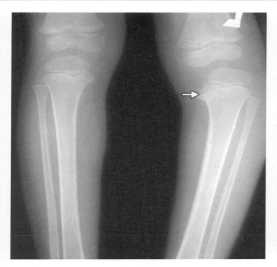

Fig. 4.83: Blount's disease (arrow).

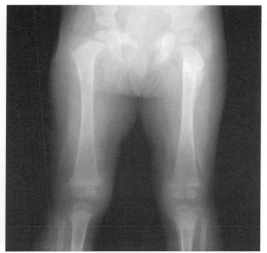

Fig. 4.84: Metadiaphyseal fractures in left femur and tibia.

weakest area (Figs. 4.84 and 4.85). The metaphyseal fracture is not associated with swelling, warmth, or pain and, therefore, not clinically apparent. Metaphyseal fractures are seen in children less than 18 months and heal slowly. In older children trauma to the metaphysis usually results in injury to the physis with complications like premature fusion or deformity. Diaphyseal fractures are fractures per se or stripped periosteum due to shearing forces. The stripped periosteum again is not clinically apparent and is seen in the X-ray as periosteal reaction after a few days. Repeated injuries like this can lead to cortical thickening.

Diaphyseal fractures are the most common. They are clinically obvious being accompanied by pain, swelling, and inability to move and, therefore, the victim is brought to the hospital. Any long bone can be fractured. If a single diaphyseal fracture is seen, there should be a search for smaller metaphyseal fractures to clinch the diagnosis of abuse. Rib fractures occur due to compression forces.

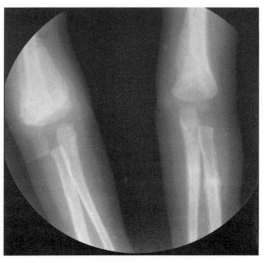

Fig. 4.85: Metadiaphyseal fractures in humerus and radius.

Multiple ribs are involved bilaterally and symmetrically (Fig. 4.86). Ribs are fractured posteriorly adjacent to the costochondral junctions or laterally at the mid-axillary lines. If road traffic accidents and fragile bones are excluded, rib fractures signify abuse. In

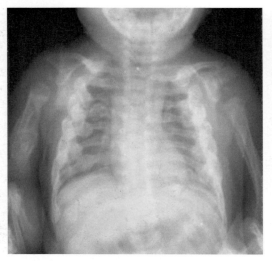

Fig. 4.86: Battered baby syndrome. Note multiple rib and humerus fractures.

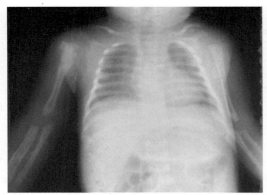

Fig. 4.87: Caffey's disease. Osteomyelitis-like features in right humerus and radius.

osteogenesis imperfecta, bones are porotic and ribs are thin and gracile. Skull fractures can also occur. Suspicious fractures include nonparietal fractures, growing fractures, and multiple fractures.

Infantile Cortical Hyperostosis

This condition of unknown etiology was first described by Caffey and hence is called Caffey's disease. It presents in infancy from as early as 2 months, but can present as late as 4 years. Clinically there is fever, irritability, and painful swellings. Radiologically there is cortical thickening and sclerosis involving one or more bones, usually multiple. The bones involved are the mandible, clavicles, scapulae, ribs, and long bones (Fig. 4.87). The pelvis may be affected, but the phalanges and vertebrae are never involved. In the mandible, the rami and coronoid process is involved but not the condyle. Involvement of the mandible clinches the diagnosis of Caffey's diseases. If a single bone is involved, diagnosis is difficult as it may be mistaken

for chronic osteomyelitis, abuse, or even malignant tumor.

Histiocytosis

Langerhans cell histiocytosis is non-neoplastic proliferation of Langerhans cells. It is of unknown etiology. There are three forms of the disease. Eosinophilic granuloma is the benign type in which skeletal manifestations predominate. It commonly presents before 10 years. The bones commonly involved are skull, spine, pelvis (Fig. 4.88), ribs, and mandible. The characteristic feature is the geographic lytic lesion seen in the calvarium (Fig. 4.89). In the jaw, there is destruction of the alveolar bone leading to floating teeth appearance (Fig. 4.90). In the spine, there is extreme wafer thin vertebral collapse called vertebra plana (Fig. 4.91). This is common in the thoracic spine, followed by lumbar spine and then cervical spine. In the long bones, there is cortical destruction resulting in lytic lesions in the metadiaphysis. Healing takes many months. The other two forms of the disease are Letterer–Siwe disease and Hand-Schüller-Christian disease. The first one is the severe acute type where there is

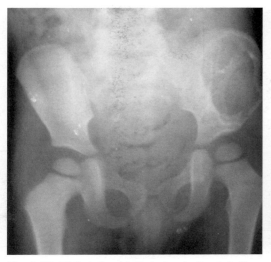

Fig. 4.88: Well-defined lytic lesion in the left ilium with a thin sclerotic border.

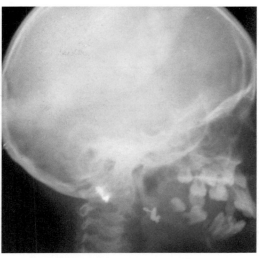

Fig. 4.90: Histiocytosis. Floating teeth appearance.

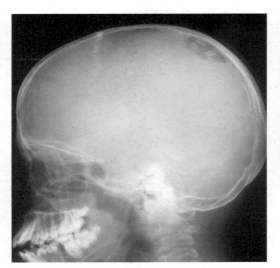

Fig. 4.89: Histiocytosis. Geographic lytic lesion in the vertex.

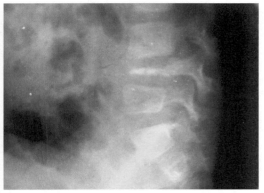

Fig. 4.91: Histiocytosis. Vertebra plana.

calvarial lesions constitute a typical triad seen in 10% of patients. Bone involvement is similar to eosinophilic granuloma.

■ SOME CONGENITAL ABNORMALITIES

Craniostenosis

hepatosplenomegaly and lymphadenopathy. These children do not live long enough to develop the skeletal manifestations. Hand-Schüller-Christian disease is as rare as the aforementioned, but runs a chronic course. Exophthalmos, diabetes insipidus, and

This is a disorder in which a single or multiple sutures undergo premature fusion causing abnormal shape of the skull and sometimes the face. Etiology is uncertain. It may be a part of Crouzon syndrome when it is associated with facial bone hypoplasia or Apert's or Carpenter's syndrome when it occurs along with syndactyly or polysyndactyly. Fusion of sutures occurring in microcephaly is not craniostenosis. In this case, the small brain does not give sufficient pressure to keep the sutures open. Premature fusion of the sagittal suture results in a skull that is elongated in the antero-posterior plane. The frontal and occipital bones compensate for the restricted lateral growth. When both the coronal sutures fuse, the result is a short skull. Plagiocephaly or asymmetric skull is due to fusion of one coronal suture (Fig. 4.92). The coronal suture is obliterated and elevation of the ipsilateral sphenoid ridge gives the orbit an upward slant called "harlequin appearance." Lambdoid synostosis causes flattening of the ipsilateral parieto-occipital region. Premature fusion of the metopic suture causes a triangular skull and hypotelorism. When all sutures are involved, it is called oxycephaly. The deformity is progressive over the period of maximal brain growth and there is increased intracranial tension.

Bifid Anterior End of Rib

Sometimes the anterior end of a rib, usually the fourth and on right, is forked giving rise to a swelling in the anterior chest wall or pain. The chest X-ray will serve to reassure the child that it is only a minor congenital abnormality (Fig. 4.93).

Sprengel Deformity

The Sprengel deformity is a congenital defect where the scapula is elevated and medially placed. It may be unilateral or bilateral. The scapula fails to descend from its fetal position. Often there is an osseous or fibrous omovertebral bar that anchors the scapula to one or more cervical vertebrae, C5, 6, or 7. In Figure 4.94, the scapula on the left is higher.

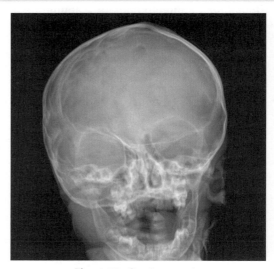

Fig. 4.92: Craniostenosis.

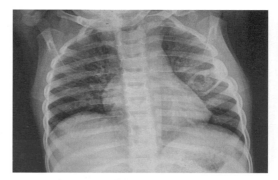

Fig. 4.93: Bifid anterior end of rib.

Klippel-Feil abnormality or renal anomalies (absence or duplication) may coexist. If the superomedial angle of the scapula is above the T2 transverse process, surgical option may be considered.

Vertebral Abnormalities

The block vertebra is seen when there is failure of separation of two adjacent vertebrae. There may be partial or complete fusion with absent or rudimentary disc space. It is usually an incidental finding and gains importance

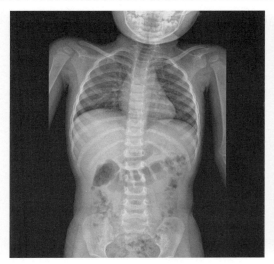

Fig. 4.94: Sprengel deformity.

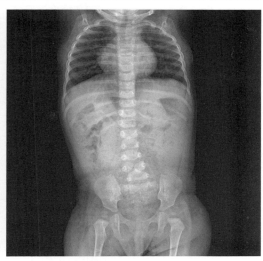

Fig. 4.95: Butterfly vertebra.

when it has to be differentiated from caries of the spine with loss of disk space. A useful point is that the height of the fused bodies equals the sum of the heights of the two vertebrae and the intervertebral disc space between them. "A waist" or mild constriction is seen at the level of the disc space between the two vertebrae. In acquired vertebral fusion, this height is less than in congenital fusion. Block vertebrae are usually seen in the cervical and lumbar spine.

Hemivertebrae occur due to lack of ossification of right or left half of the vertebral body. Scoliosis is present at birth. Butterfly vertebrae (Fig. 4.95) occur when the right and left halves do not unite. Vertebral abnormalities are seen as part of the VACTERL complex (Fig. 4.96). They often accompany neurenteric or duplication cysts. This is due to their close embryologic relationship. The notochord, which is at first fused with the embryonic endoderm, separates from it. If separation is incomplete traction, diverticulae and duplication cysts develop.

Widening of the spinal canal with spreading of the pedicles is a feature of

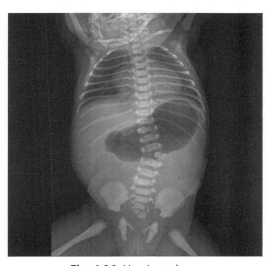

Fig. 4.96: Hemivertebrae.

posterior meningocele. Soft tissue shadow of the meningocele is seen overlying the spine.

Developmental Dysplasia of the Hip

In this condition, there is abnormal development of the acetabulum, which is shallow and therefore does not hold the femoral head that is dislocated. Routine clinical

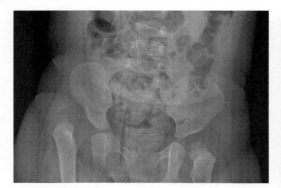

Fig. 4.97: Developmental dysplasia of hip.

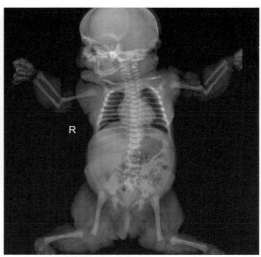

Fig. 4.98: Arthrogryposis multiplex.

examination is mandatory to pick up DDH in the newborn period as early treatment is essential for good results. Ultrasound is a very useful modality for this. In the newborn and young infant, the head of the femur is entirely cartilaginous and not visualized in the X-ray. Hence, certain lines are used to aid diagnosis. A horizontal line drawn through both triradiate cartilage is called the Hilgenreiner line. The Perkin's line is a vertical line dropped from the outer edge of the acetabulum. Normally, the head of the femur or the supero-medial edge of the metaphysis lies in the lower inner quadrant (Fig. 4.97). In dislocation, it lies in the upper outer quadrant.

Arthrogryposis Multiplex Congenital

This is a large group of genetic disorders characterized by multiple joint contractures present at birth. The muscles of the affected limbs are hypoplastic and the muscle plane in the X-ray is lucent like the subcutaneous fat. There are multiple dislocations (Fig. 4.98). Amyoplasia is the severe form with extensive involvement of limbs while distal arthrogryposis mainly involves the distal parts of limbs.

Gastrointestinal System

TK Nandakumaran

CONVENTIONAL X-RAY OF ABDOMEN IN INFANTS AND CHILDREN

With the advancement in technology, X-ray of abdomen, as a diagnostic tool, has been pushed to a lower level and modalities like ultrasonography, CT scan, and MRI have attained priority. Still in infants and children, a lot of information can be obtained by conventional X-ray. In fact, many neonatal abdominal conditions can be diagnosed by conventional X-ray alone. Air in the gastrointestinal tract is a good contrast medium. In relevant cases, other contrast material like Barium (Ba) or gastrografin can be used. The timing and position of the child during X-ray is important. Air enters the stomach within few minutes, small bowel in 3 hours and sigmoid colon in 9 hours. Air also rises to the uppermost part of the peritoneal cavity.

X-ray in erect posture gives most useful information. Lateral decubitus position is also useful. Chest must always be included with abdominal X-ray. Chest conditions like pneumonia mimic acute abdomen.

Gasless abdomen: Indicates a baby with pure esophageal atresia without tracheoesophageal fistula.

GASTRIC OUTLET OBSTRUCTION

Pyloric Atresia and Pyloric Membrane

Both presents in the immediate newborn period as nonbile stained vomiting. Other symptoms include excessive salivation and respiratory problems. Abdomen is not distended. Epigastric fullness or visible gastric peristalsis may be present. Plain radiography is diagnostic. Air acts as a good contrast medium. If there is fluid in the stomach, the fluid is aspirated and some air is instilled. Barium contrast is rarely required (Figs. 5.1 and 5.2). Single large stomach bubble is found. No air extends beyond pylorus. Given time, single large air fluid level will be seen.

Infantile Hypertrophic Pyloric Stenosis

It affects first-born male child in 80%. Non-bile stained vomiting, onset between 2 and 8

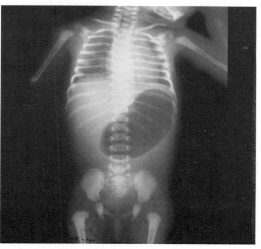

Fig. 5.1: Plain X-ray of pyloric atresia. Note single large stomach bubble. No other air shadow is seen.

weeks, vomits soon after feeds, which is persistent and later becomes projectile. Voracious appetite, take feeds immediately after vomiting. Constipation, dehydration, and visible gastric peristalsis are other clinical features. Small pyloric mass to the size of tip of little finger may be palpated.

Barium meal study shows elongated pyloric channel with shoulders proximally with indirect evidence of pyloric muscle hypertrophy. Small amount of contrast in the duodenal bulb define the length of pyloric canal (String sign of Cantor).

■ DUODENAL OBSTRUCTION

It occurs in 1 in 6,000–7,000 livebirths. 50% mothers have polyhydramnios and 50% of the babies are premature. Congenital anomalies in other organ systems are seen in 50% of cases.

One-third of cases are associated with Down syndrome. Bile stained vomiting within few hours after birth is the most common presentation. Fullness in the epigastrium due to dilated stomach or visible gastric peristalsis is seen. Rest of the abdomen is scaphoid. Meconium not passed in total obstruction. Clinical spectra include the following:

❏ Duodenal atresia
❏ Duodenal web
❏ Annular pancreas
❏ Duodenal diaphragm
❏ Malrotation.

■ DUODENAL ATRESIA

Plain X-ray of the abdomen in the erect posture is usually characteristic. There is loss of continuity of the lumen, distal to the second part of duodenum. Distension of the stomach and duodenum gives rise to the classical double bubble sign (Fig. 5.3). Bubble on the left side is due to air fluid level in the stomach and bubble on the right side is due to air fluid level in the distended duodenum. This finding may be obscured if there is plenty of fluid. In such situation, the

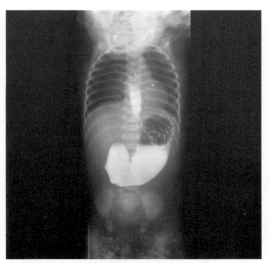

Fig. 5.2: Barium meal contrast of pyloric atresia. Stomach is filled with barium. No barium beyond pylorus is seen.

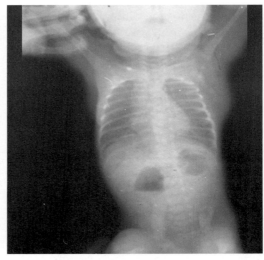

Fig. 5.3: Double bubble sign.

fluid should be aspirated and 60 mL of air should be injected. This is pathognomonic of duodenal atresia. There is no gas beyond the second part of duodenum. This picture is also seen in duodenal web.

ANNULAR PANCREAS AND DUODENAL DIAPHRAGM

It causes incomplete duodenal obstruction. Signs and symptoms are similar as in duodenal atresia, but meconium is passed. It may present beyond infancy. In addition to this, there may be associated atresia or stenosis at the same level. Plain X-ray shows dilated stomach and duodenum (double bubble). There is paucity of air shadow in the abdomen. Barium meal will show dilated stomach and duodenal bulb and specks of barium in the distal bowel (Fig. 5.4).

MALROTATION OF THE BOWEL

It includes various clinical presentations, ranging from chronic abdominal pain to midgut volvulus. Primary presenting sign of malrotation is sudden onset of bilious vomiting. Lower abdomen appears scaphoid. When there is volvulus and ischemic insult, there is sudden deterioration of general condition and abdominal distension. Plain X-ray may not be contributory; sometimes there may be dilated stomach. Barium (Ba) meal study is classical. Duodenal C loop is not formed. Normally duodenum forms a "C" loop, goes to the left of vertebral column and continuous as jejunum at the level of L1 vertebrae (Fig. 5.5). In malrotation, instead jejunum starts on the right side (Fig. 5.6).

JEJUNAL ATRESIA

It includes more than two gas bubbles in the upper abdomen, not multiple air fluid level as in lower intestinal obstruction. Distal most part of atretic segment shows bulbous dilation. No gas is present in lower part of abdomen.

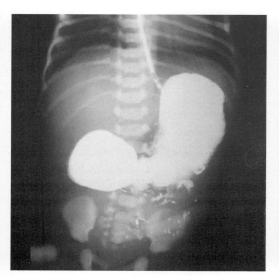

Fig. 5.4: Barium meal showing dilated stomach and duodenal bulb.

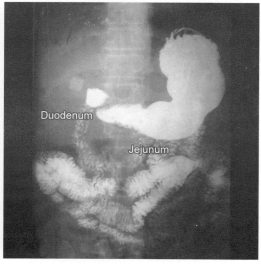

Fig. 5.5: Normal barium meal study.

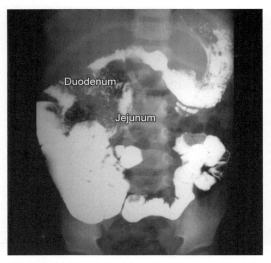

Fig. 5.6: Malrotation: Jejunum starts on the right side.

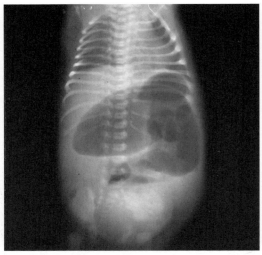

Fig. 5.7: Jejunal atresia: Multiple air fluid level in the upper abdomen. No gas in lower abdomen.

■ ILEAL ATRESIA

Incidence of this condition is 1 in 1,500 livebirths. 50% of them have low birth weight. These babies will have bilious vomiting, abdominal distension, and failure to pass meconium. Diagnosis is usually confirmed by plain X-ray.

High jejunal atresia is present with few air fluid levels and no further gas beyond that is present (Fig. 5.7). The more distal is the atresia, the greater is the number of air fluid levels (Fig. 5.8).

Meconium Ileus

Bilious vomiting and failure to pass meconium is the usual presentation. When there are complications, like perforation, they will present with features of peritonitis (Fig. 5.9).

Giant Cyst Meconium Peritonitis

Intrauterine perforation causes sterile peritonitis and escape of air and subsequent encystation causes this condition (Fig. 5.10).

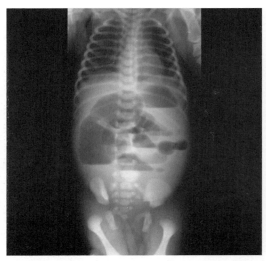

Fig. 5.8: Proximal ileal atresia: Multiple air fluid level in the upper two-thirds of the abdomen. No gas in lower abdomen. Note the bulbous dilation of distal most part of the proximal bowel.

Microcolon

It can be seen in any condition where meconium has not entered the colon. Example

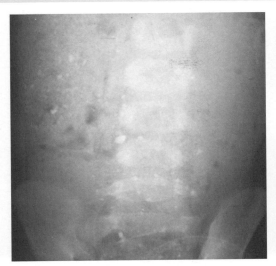

Fig. 5.9: Meconium ileus. Note the ground glass appearance due to the mixing of air and meconium. Multiple calcification is peculiar to meconium ileus.

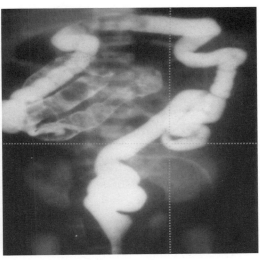

Fig. 5.11: Barium enema. Colon is uniformly narrow throughout. Note the barium in terminal ileum.

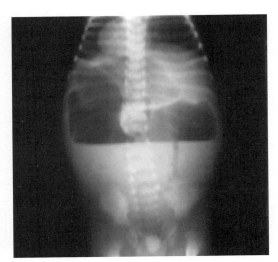

Fig. 5.10: Meconium peritonitis. Note the unusually large air fluid level.

includes jejunoileal atresia, meconium ileus, and total colonic aganglionosis (Fig. 5.11).

■ HIRSCHSPRUNG'S DISEASE

This disease affects 1 in 5,000 newborn babies. Male to female ratio is 4:1. It is present with delay in passing meconium in first 24 hours, abdominal distension, and vomiting. There is absence of ganglion cells in the submucus and myenteric plexus. Aganglionic segment fails to relax, thereby causing functional obstruction to the propulsion of fecal matter. Plain X-ray shows distended bowel loops throughout the abdomen. It is difficult to identify colon and ileum in newborn X-ray (Fig. 5.12).

Barium Enema in Hirschsprung's Disease

Rectal examination and washout should be avoided because it will distort the transition zone. Catheter should be inserted just inside the anus. Slow hand injection is done with slow and steady pressure. Undue pressure will distort the picture.

Classical findings include spastic distal intestinal segment with dilated proximal colon (Fig. 5.13). Normally rectum is more dilated than sigmoid. In Hirschsprung's

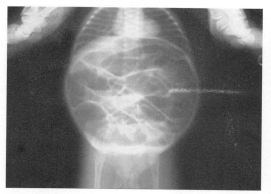

Fig. 5.12: Hirschsprung's disease. Note the distended bowel loops.

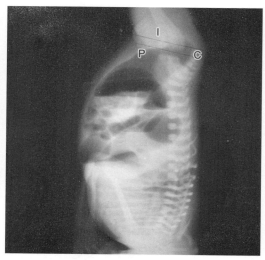

Fig. 5.14: Low anomaly.

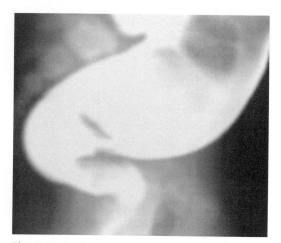

Fig. 5.13: Barium enema in Hirschsprung's disease showing narrow rectum and dilated sigmoid.

disease (HD), rectum is narrow, sigmoid is dilated. Normally, rectosigmoid index (ratio of the diameter of rectum to sigmoid) is more than 1. In HD, it is less than 1.

◼ ANORECTAL MALFORMATIONS

These malformations occur in 1 in 5,000 livebirths. There is slight male preponderance. Low lesions are indicated more in females. Associated anomalies are common.

Management of this condition depends on assessing whether lesion is high, intermediate, or low. For this, invertogram or prone lateral view is taken. Invertogram is taken 24 hours after birth so that air will reach the distal most end of the bowel. Prone lateral-ray also is taken after the same period. X-ray is interpreted depending on the bony landmark and air contrast.

Bony points marked are as follows:

P—Pubic bone (center of pubic bone)

C—Coccyx (last piece of sacrum (because coccyx is not ossified in newborns)

I—Ischium (lower most point of ischial bone)

Lines drawn are as follows:

PC line—connecting pubic bone and coccyx. I line—parallel line through lowermost point of the ischial bone.

Air shadow going beyond I line is low anomaly (Figs. 5.14 and 5.15), gas shadow between PC and I line is intermediate anomaly (Fig. 5.16) and gas shadow proximal to PC line is high anomaly (Fig. 5.17).

Ascites

Its causes include chylous, biliary, urinary, pancreatic, etc. Whole abdomen is hazy and only few gas bubbles will be seen (Fig. 5.18).

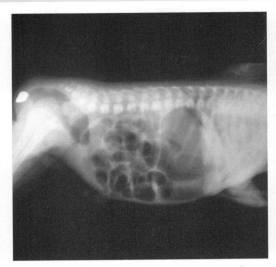

Fig. 5.15: Prone lateral view. Low anomaly.

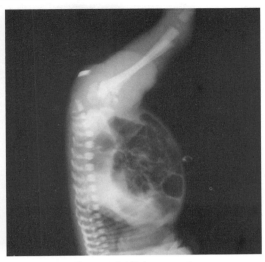

Fig. 5.17: High anomaly.

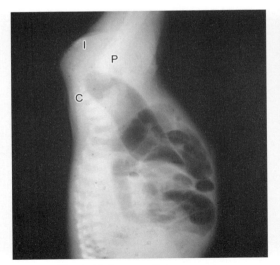

Fig. 5.16: Intermediate anomaly.

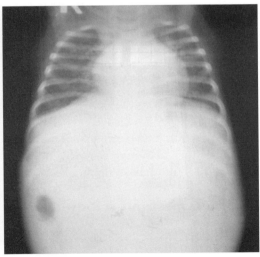

Fig. 5.18: Ascites: abdomen is hazy.

Congenital Diaphragmatic Hernia

❑ Bochdalek hernia (posterolateral defect is the most common type)

❑ Morgagni hernia (central defect).

Its incidence is 1 in 5,000 livebirths. Left posterolateral defect is found in 80% of cases, 20% right sided. Most of them present in the newborn period with respiratory distress. Few cases are present in infancy and childhood with recurrent respiratory infection. Diagnosis is done by plain X-ray of abdomen and chest in the erect posture. Features include absence of diaphragmatic

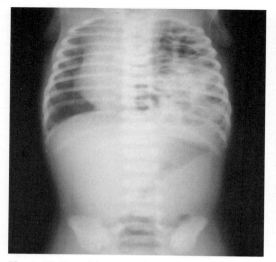

Fig. 5.19: Bowel loops in the chest. Note the paucity of gas shadow in the abdomen.

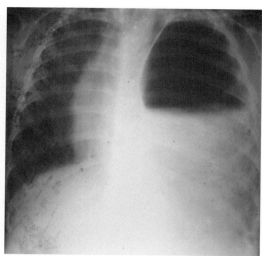

Fig. 5.20: Diaphragmatic hernia: Mimicking hydropneumothorax.

dome, bowel shadow continuous with the shadow in the chest, shift of mediastinum to opposite side and paucity of gas shadow in the abdomen. A Ryle's tube will help to locate the stomach in the chest (Fig. 5.19).

Differential Diagnosis

It includes congenital cystic adenomatoid malformation, pneumatocele, agenesis of lung, and eventration of diaphragm.

Diaphragmatic Hernia in Older Children

Children presents with recurrent respiratory tract infection. Beware of the hydropneumothorax on left side. Before putting a chest tube, a Ryle's tube must be put and an X-ray should be taken (Figs. 5.20 and 5.21). This X-ray shows air fluid level in left chest. Carefully look at the smooth dome over the gas shadow, which is an indication for the presence of diaphragm (Fig. 5.22). The Ryle's tube in chest cavity in the same patient can be seen.

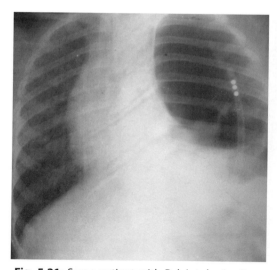

Fig. 5.21: Same patient with Ryle's tube in situ.

Morgagni Hernia

It includes less than 2% of diaphragmatic defect. It is usually seen in older children and adult. It is a herniation through sterna and costal attachment of diaphragm. Sac is present and colon or small bowel is the

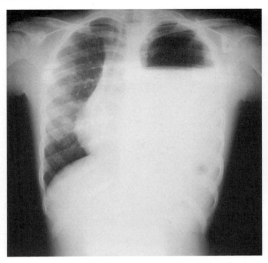

Fig. 5.22: Same patient as in Figure 5.21. Barium meal X-ray. Note the barium filling the stomach in chest and paucity of gas shadow in the abdomen.

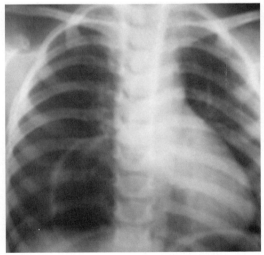

Fig. 5.23: Barium meal followed through X-ray in Morgagni hernia. Note the colon inside the chest.

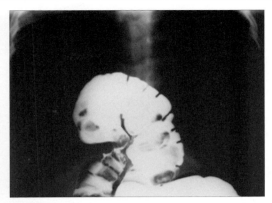

Fig. 5.24: Morgagni hernia: Barium study.

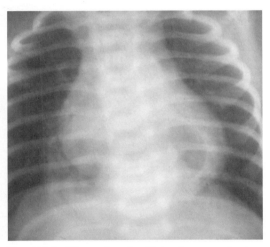

Fig. 5.25: Hiatus hernia. Note the gas shadow within the mediastinum.

Hiatus Hernia

Rare type of hernia in children often present in older age group. Plain X-ray may show air in the mediastinum (Fig. 5.25). Barium studies will confirm the diagnosis (Fig. 5.26).

Eventration of Diaphragm

❑ Diaphragm is thin and membranous
❑ Muscle deficiency in diaphragm is found
❑ Diaphragm is pushed into the chest (Fig. 5.27).

content. Radiograph shows a mass or air fluid level in chest radiograph just above diaphragm. Barium study is confirmatory (Figs. 5.23 and 5.24). Note encysted air space above diaphragm and mediastinum.

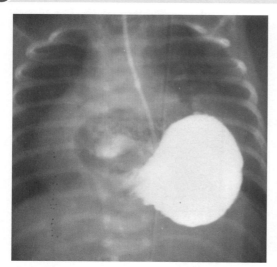

Fig. 5.26: Barium filling the cystic lesion in the mediastinum.

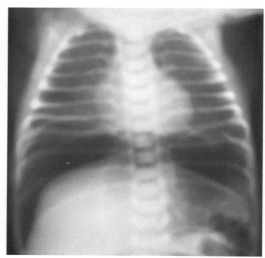

Fig. 5.28: Pneumoperitoneum—drooping lily appearance.

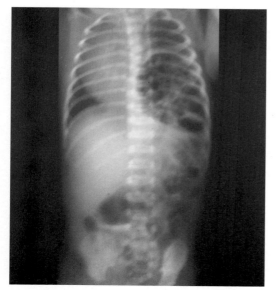

Fig. 5.27: Eventration of diaphragm. Note the mediastinal diaphragmatic contour on the left side of the chest.

- Diaphragmatic contour is seen.
- Immobility of diaphragm is demonstrated by fluoroscopy.

Pneumoperitoneum

There is gas under diaphragm. Liver, stomach, and spleen are separated from diaphragm by intervening gas—drooping lily appearance (Fig. 5.28).

Pure Esophageal Atresia

It includes gasless abdomen. Due to esophageal atresia, baby cannot swallow air (Fig. 5.29).

Achalasia Cardia

It is present with dysphagia, more for liquids than solids. Dilated esophagus with tapering lower end is present. Small stomach is indicated (Fig. 5.30).

Intussusception

It occurs in infants of 3–9 months. It is usually present with incessant cry, vomiting, passing blood, and mucus per rectum, sausage-shaped mass in the abdomen.

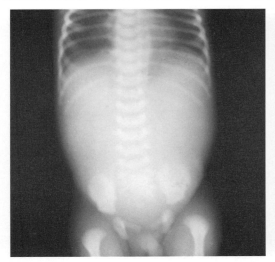

Fig. 5.29: Pure esophageal atresia: Gasless abdomen.

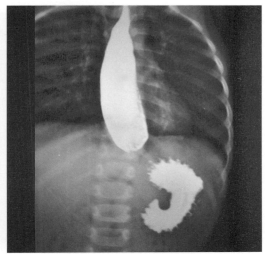

Fig. 5.30: Dilated esophagus with tapering lower end—a case of achalasia cardia.

Barium Enema X-ray

It indicates cut of sign at the site of mass, claw sign as the barium fills the apex of intussusception (Fig. 5.31). Coiled spring appearance in loose intussusceptions barium fills between the loops of intussusception.

Abdominopelvic Cyst

Whole of intestine is pushed to the upper abdomen. Lower half of the abdomen shows haziness (Fig. 5.32).

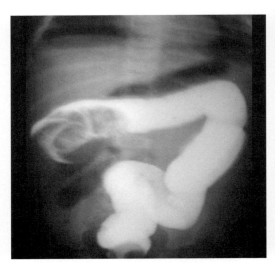

Fig. 5.31: Claw sign in intussusception.

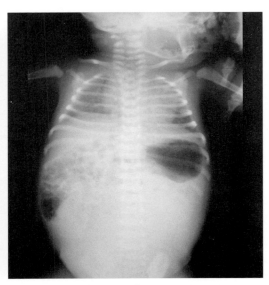

Fig. 5.32: Abdominopelvic cyst. Intestines are pushed upward.

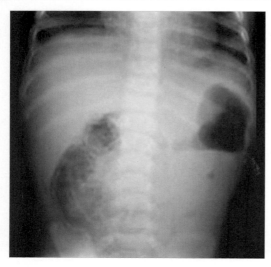

Fig. 5.33: Necrotizing enterocolitis. Note gas shadow upward in the intestinal wall.

Pneumatosis Intestinalis

It is seen in necrotizing enterocolitis, enterocolitis of Hirschsprung's disease, inspissated milk syndrome, severe diarrhea and carbohydrate intolerance, etc. (Fig. 5.33).

Genitourinary System

Anand S Vasudev, Manish Kumar

▌ CONVENTIONAL RADIOLOGY IN PEDIATRIC RENAL DISEASES

Imaging plays a major role in evaluation of suspected renal diseases in pediatric patients. Conventional radiology includes plain X-rays of abdomen, voiding cystourethrogram (VCUG) and intravenous urography (IVU). Last decade has seen a major revolution in imaging techniques of renal diseases with introduction of ultrasonography (USG), computerized tomography (CT) scan, magnetic resonance imaging (MRI), and nuclear imaging. Although, newer advanced imaging modalities provide better structural and functional details, conventional radiology remains a valuable tool, alone or in combination, in certain specific renal diseases like renal stones, spinal abnormalities leading to neurogenic bladder, vesicoureteral reflux (VUR), and congenital structural malformation of the kidneys. Choice of imaging technique depends on type of renal disease, availability of technique, cost, requirement of sedation, radiation exposure, and risk of contrast administration.

Role of conventional radiology has diminished with the introduction of newer imaging technology. However, importance of plain radiography, VCUG, and IVU cannot be denied in evaluation of specific renal diseases and assessment of renal function, particularly in resource poor areas. X-ray abdomen: Plain

X-ray of abdomen is the oldest modality of radiological investigation. Imaging of urinary tract starts with conventional radiograph of the kidney, ureter, and bladder, commonly called a "KUB" film (Fig. 6.1). Apart from a very few clinical conditions, this is rarely used as a primary investigative modality in evaluation of renal diseases. Sometimes, fecalith may appear as calcified structure in bladder mimicking stones (Fig. 6.2).

Indications

❏ As a scout film for other procedures, like IVU and VCUG, before contrast

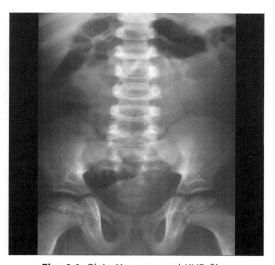

Fig. 6.1: Plain X-ray normal KUB film.

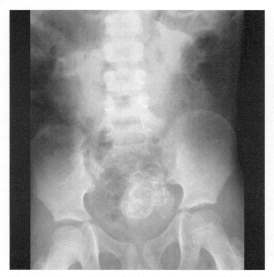

Fig. 6.2: X-ray of KUB (kidney, ureter, and bladder) showing fecalith.

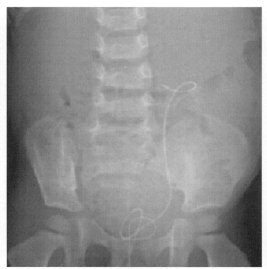

Fig. 6.3: X-ray of KUB (kidney, ureter, and bladder) showing migration of stent from its normal position.

administration, so not to obscure radio-paque stones and calcified structures

☐ Suspected renal or bladder stones
☐ To assess correct positioning and migration of various drainage catheters and stents (Fig. 6.3)
☐ Neurogenic bladder to evaluate spinal deformities (Figs. 6.4A to C).

Technique

A "KUB" film is usually taken after a good bowel preparation to minimize the effect of feces and bowel gases and taken on empty stomach. X-ray is usually obtained in supine position at the end of full expiration. Upper margin of the X-ray should contain suprarenal areas and lower margin should include pubic rami. Lateral views are obtained if spinal deformity is noted.

Normal renal outlines can be seen unless they are obscured by bowel gases. Ureter is usually not visualized unless a calculus is present, which can be seen along the course of the ureter. Presence of vertebral scoliosis or obliteration of normal psoas shadow may suggest renal or pararenal inflammation (Figs. 6.4A to C).

■ UROLITHIASIS

Most of the urinary tract calculi are radiopaque and so easily visible on X-ray KUB. Radiolucent stones, such as uric acid stones, cannot be detected on plain X-ray, but may appear as filling defect within the opacified urinary tract on IVU or may be visualized in ultrasonologic examination. X-ray can demonstrate exact number, size, and location of urinary tract calculi (Figs. 6.5 and 6.6). Staghorn calculi can be easily diagnosed on X-ray KUB. Nephrocalcinosis can be detected incidentally on X-ray KUB. However, because of easy availability and absence of ionizing radiation USG is the modality of choice for detecting urolithiasis and nephrocalcinosis.

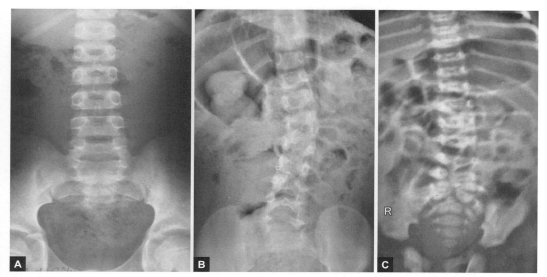

Figs. 6.4A to C: Plain X-ray of abdomen showing spinal deformities. (A) Spina bifida S1; (B) Scoliosis with segmentation anomalies of lumbar and sacral vertebrae in case of neurogenic bladder; (C) Segmentation anomalies of lumbar and sacral vertebrae.

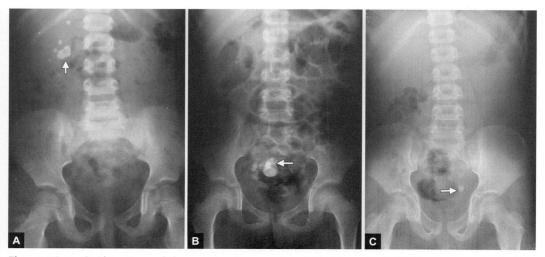

Figs. 6.5A to C: Plain X-ray abdomen showing renal and bladder calculi. (A) Multiple renal calculi in right pelvicalyceal system; (B) A large vesical calculus with multiple small calculi; (C) A calculus at left vesicoureteric junction.

Intravenous Urography

Historically, IVU has been the investigation of choice for defining anatomical details and function of the upper urinary tract. With advancement in imaging technique, use of IVU has decreased considerably, especially in children due to its high radiation dose, but

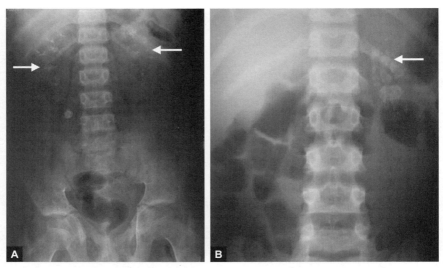

Figs. 6.6A and B: (A) X-ray KUB showing bilateral nephrocalcinosis; (B) X-ray KUB showing calcium deposits in left kidney.

it still remains an excellent tool for a number of clinical conditions. It provides excellent anatomical details in many congenital urinary tract anomalies. In resource-limited areas, IVU still remains the investigation of choice in the evaluation of urolithiasis, hydronephrosis, and detection of renal scars. As result of IVU depends on functioning of the kidneys, quality of anatomic information is often compromised and delayed in cases of compromised renal function. It also cannot provide information on parenchymal structure and estimation of glomerular filtration rate (GFR) when the renal functions are not adequate. Use of contrast and ionizing radiation also limits its use in pediatric practice.

Preparation

Bowel preparation is done night before IVU by using good laxative. Patient is normally kept nil per orally 5–6 hours before the procedure. An adequate hydration is maintained.

Technique

A KUB film is taken before injection of contrast agent to assess bowel preparation and to detect any radio-opaque stone, vertebral anomaly or any calcified structure. After injecting the contrast a series of films are taken at 1-, 5-, 10-, 15-, and 30-minute intervals (Figs. 6.7A to E). Number of films varies from one institution to other and depends on clinical diagnosis of the patient. One- and five-minute films are taken centered on the kidneys with appropriate gonad shield to show the nephrogram and pelvicalyceal system. Subsequent films (10, 15, and 30 minutes) are full-length films to show the ureter and urinary bladder. Delayed films are taken for the evaluation of obstructive uropathy.

Indications

1. *Urolithiasis*: USG is the most commonly used test for the diagnosis of renal calculi. However, it often fails to detect ureteric

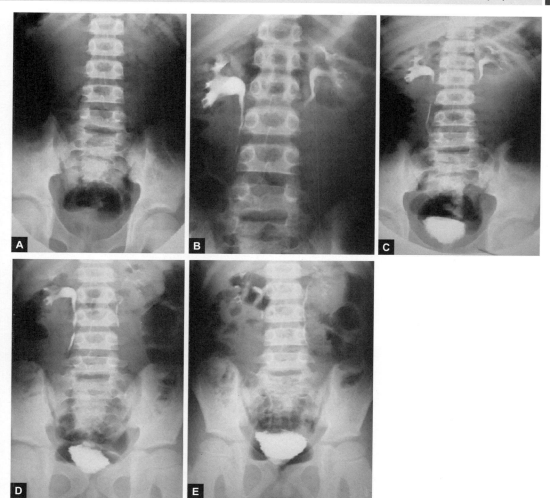

Figs. 6.7A to E: Normal IVP. (A) Control film; (B) 5-minute film showing prompt uptake and excretion of radiocontrast by both the kidneys, normal pelvicalyceal system; (C) 10-minute film showing normal excretion by both the kidneys; (D) 15-minute film; (E) 30-minute film showing complete excretion of radiocontrast by both the kidneys.

calculi. Sensitivity of nonhelical CT scan is better than USG in detecting renal stones. IVU helps in identifying exact number, size, and location of the stones (Figs. 6.8A to D). It also detects hydro-nephrosis secondary to obstruction if any and helps in evaluation of renal function (Figs. 6.9A to C).

2. *Congenital kidney and urological disorders*: IVU is most commonly used modality to assess congenital urinary tract anomaly, alone or in combination with other investigations.

3. *Renal agenesis*: Bilateral renal agenesis is the most severe developmental anomaly of the urinary tract, with an incidence of 1–3

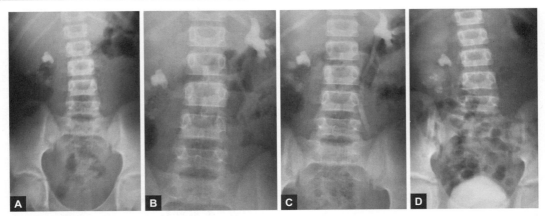

Figs. 6.8A to D: Intravenous urography showing right-sided obstructed hydronephrosis due to renal calculi. (A) Scout film shows right staghorn calculus with multiple small calculi at lower pole of right kidney; (B) 10-minute film shows prompt uptake and excretion by the left kidney showing normal pelvicalyceal system on the left side and dense nephrogram on the left side; (C) 15-minute film shows normal left ureter draining into the bladder. Right kidney is severely hydronephrotic and right ureter is not visualized; (D) Delayed film (1 hour) shows hold up of the radiocontrast material and enlarged right kidney suggestive of hydronephrosis.

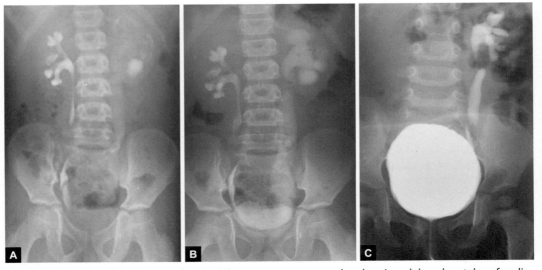

Figs. 6.9A to C: Hydroureteronephrosis. (A) Intravenous urography showing delayed uptake of radio-contrast material in left hydronephrotic kidney with dense nephrogram; (B) Left dilated pelvicalyceal system and dilated ureter; (C) Delayed excretion of radiocontrast material from hydronephrotic left kidney.

per 10,000 live births. The condition can be diagnosed by antenatal sonography as severe oligohydramnios, absence of fetal bladder, and both kidneys. Conventional radiology has no role in diagnosis of bilateral renal agenesis. Unilateral renal agenesis occurs with an incidence of 1 per 1,000 live births, predominantly in males and on the left side. The condition can be diagnosed with antenatal USG or as an incidental USG finding done for some other reason. IVU is usually advised to differentiate it from an ectopic kidney, which can be located anywhere along the course of renal ascent. However, poor renal function may limit the sensitivity to detect ectopic kidney by IVU.

4. *Uncrossed ectopic kidney and malrotated kidney*: Ectopic kidney results from failure of ascent of normal kidney from pelvis to its normal position during early fetal life and can be seen lying anywhere along its path of ascent. The condition is normally diagnosed with USG. IVU is generally advised to confirm the abnormal position of the kidney with malrotation, if any, and associated problems like obstruction (Figs. 6.10 and 6.11).

5. *Crossed fused renal ectopia*: This condition results when kidney of one side crosses the midline and fuses with the opposite side kidney. Incidence of this condition is 1 in 1,000–2,000 per live births. Malrotation with other abnormalities like pelviureteric junction (PUJ) obstruction and reflux is frequently seen in the ectopic kidney. Although, USG may demonstrate unusually large kidney on the affected side with absent kidney on the opposite side, IVU establishes the diagnosis and clearly delineates the anatomy of the urinary tract (Fig. 6.12).

6. *Horseshoe kidney*: The horseshoe kidney is the most frequent renal fusion anomaly and occurs 1 per 400 people. The condition results from fusion of lower pole of both the kidneys across the midline in early fetal life. Kidney lies lower than normal

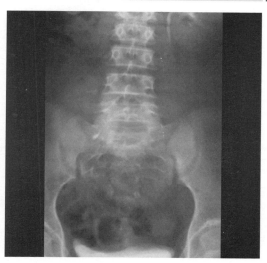

Fig. 6.10: Ectopic right kidney. Intravenous urography shows normal left kidney. Right kidney is absent in right renal fossa and is present in right lumbosacral region, seen as dense nephrogram over right side of L4, L5, and right sacroiliac joint. Right kidney is functioning normally as evidenced by normal contrast excretion and right ureter is draining normally into urinary bladder.

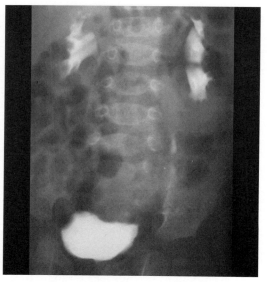

Fig. 6.11: Left-sided malrotated kidney. Intravenous urography shows anteriorly rotated left-sided pelvicalyceal system.

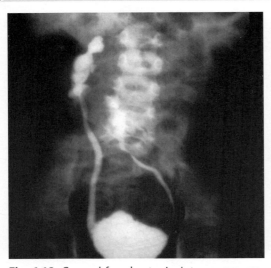

Fig. 6.12: Crossed fused ectopia. Intravenous urography showing left kidney crossing over and fusing with lower pole of right kidney. Left ureter crosses the midline and opens at its normal site.

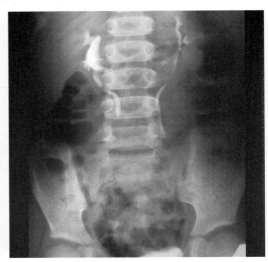

Fig. 6.13: Horseshoe kidney. Intravenous urography showing lower pole of both the kidneys directed medially and ureter passing over the anterior aspect of the vertebrae.

position anterior to aorta and inferior vena cava and pelvicalyceal system face anteriorly. Associated abnormalities like PUJ obstruction and reflux are frequently seen (Fig. 6.13).

Intravenous urography typically shows U-shaped nephrogram with lower calyces moving medially, resulting in "hand-holding calyces" appearance. The lower calyces are often medial to the ipsilateral ureter. PUJ or UVJ obstruction can be seen as an associated finding.

7. *Duplex kidney:* A duplex kidney results from two separate pelvicalyceal systems in one kidney. The two ureters may join somewhere along their course or may open separately in the urinary bladder. According to Weigert-Mayer rule, the upper ureter joins the bladder more medially and inferiorly to the orifice of lower moiety ureter (Fig. 6.14A). Ureterocele is the frequent associated finding with upper moiety and reflux with lower

moiety ureter. USG can easily establish the diagnosis of duplex kidney; IVU is required for better delineation of morphology and functioning of duplex kidney. Often there is no or poor functioning of upper moiety kidney. Nonfilling of the obstructed upper moiety results in the downward displacement of the lower pole calyces causing the "drooping lily sign". Associated hydronephrosis secondary to PUJ or UVJ obstruction can also be seen (Fig. 6.14B).

8. *Pelviureteric junction obstruction:* PUJ obstruction is the most common cause of neonatal hydronephrosis and a major cause of obstructive uropathy at all ages. Newborns and infants usually present with palpable abdominal lump, whereas older children commonly present with flank pain, hematuria, or urinary tract infection (UTI). USG is the investigation of choice in diagnosis of PUJ obstruction in association with DTPA nuclear scan. IVU

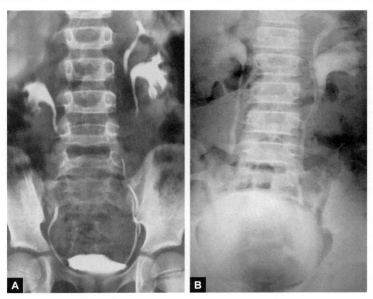

Figs. 6.14A and B: Duplex kidney. (A) Intravenous urography (IVU) showing two separate pelvicalyceal systems on the left side. Both the moieties appear to be functioning normally and the two ureters drain separately into the bladder; (B) IVU showing complete duplex system on the left side. Lower moiety shows dilatation of pelvicalyceal system suggestive of mild hydronephrosis.

classically shows delayed opacification of collecting system, dilated renal pelvis out of proportion to calyces with abrupt narrowing at junction with ureter, non-visualization of normal ureter and hold up of contrast in the pelvicalyceal system in delayed films. In severe cases nephrogenic phase of the urogram may show an opaque rim of functioning parenchyma of various thicknesses peripherally with multiple centrally placed radiolucencies representing dilated calyces, termed as a "rim sign" (Figs. 6.15 and 6.16).

The condition needs to be differentiated from prominent extra renal pelvis, where contrast appears promptly in the collecting system, calyces appear normal with sharp fornices, ureter is visualized normal without any abrupt narrowing at PUJ and prompt clearing of contrast in delayed films.

Ectopic ureter: Ectopic ureter results when a ureter fails to open at its normal superolateral aspect of bladder trigone. It is more common in female and it opens either in urethra, vestibule, or vagina. It clinically presents with continuous leakage of urine in a female with normal voiding pattern. The condition is more commonly associated with duplex kidney where upper ureter moiety opens ectopically. IVU is the investigation of choice in diagnosis of ectopic ureter opening at urethra or vagina.

Ureterocele: Ureterocele is a congenital condition characterized by cystic dilatation of the intravesical portion of the distal end of the ureter. It can be simple or ectopic. Simple ureterocele lies within the bladder (Figs. 6.17 and 6.18), whereas, ectopic ureterocele extends up to bladder neck or urethra. It is more commonly seen in upper

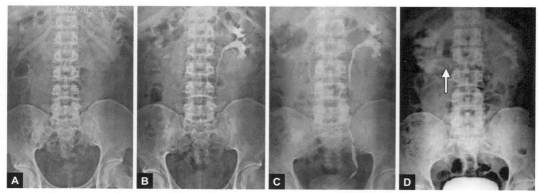

Figs. 6.15A to D: Pelviureteric junction obstruction. (A) 1-minute intravenous urography (IVU) film showing bilateral good nephrogram; (B and C) 5-minute and 15-minute IVU film respectively showing prompt excretion of radiocontrast from left kidney. Right kidney shows opaque rim of functioning parenchyma with multiple central translucencies suggestive of dilated calyces, termed as "rim sign"; (D) Delayed film (2 hours) shows hold up of contrast and dilated renal pelvis in the right kidney out of proportion to calyces with abrupt narrowing at the junction with the ureter.

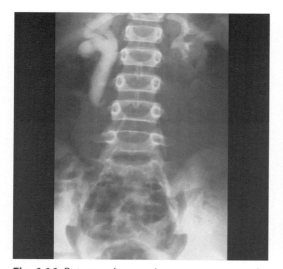

Fig. 6.16: Retrocaval ureter. Intravenous urography showing dilatation of renal pelvis and upper ureter with abrupt narrowing and kinking at T3-T4 junction suggestive of retrocaval ureter.

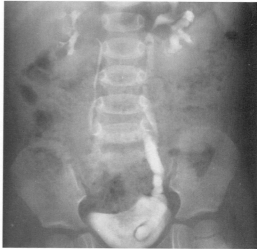

Fig. 6.17: Simple ureterocele. Intravenous urography showing a radiolucent halo representing the nonopacified wall of ureterocele, seen as "cobra head" appearance with dilatation of left ureter.

ureteric moiety of duplex kidney. USG is the most common modality of diagnosing ureterocele. IVU finding of ureterocele is very characteristic, showing as a filling defect at the distal end of the ureter, characteristic "cobra head appearance." It also delineates the anatomy of the urinary tract and helps in evaluating renal function. IVU is also used for

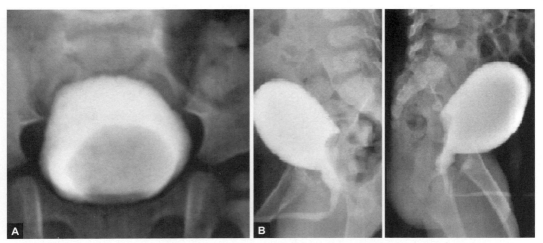

Figs. 6.18A and B: Ureterocele. (A) Voiding cystourethrogram showing filling defect in contrast filled bladder; (B) Oblique film shows filling defect in bladder suggestive of ureterocele.

preoperative assessment in renal transplant donors. Postoperative assessment, especially after pyeloplasty in PUJ obstruction, is done to look for efficacy of surgery.

Voiding Cystourethrogram

Voiding cystourethrogram is the investigation of choice in diagnosis and grading of VUR. This investigation is often labeled as micturating cystourethrogram (MCU). It also provides anatomical details of bladder and urethra (Figs. 6.19 and 6.20). It is commonly advised after an episode of UTI to detect reflux, antenatally detected hydronephrosis, suspected case of bladder outlet obstruction, anterior and posterior urethral valve (PUV), in work up of cases with chronic kidney disease and in cases with congenital urinary tract abnormalities in combination with other investigations. Sometimes, urethral stones may be detected as a filling defect in contrast filled anterior urethra (Figs. 6.21A to C).

Technique

Voiding cystourethrogram is commonly done after an episode of UTI has been treated adequately and under antibiotic coverage of oral amoxicillin or injection gentamicin. Bladder is catheterized with a feeding tube under all aseptic precaution and urine is drained out. Sedation is usually not required except in very apprehensive child. A water-soluble contrast is instilled into the bladder per urethra by a disposable syringe under fluoroscopic guidance. Volume of contrast is determined according to bladder capacity or till the child expresses a desire to void.

Bladder capacity is calculated as:
- In child under 1 year of age, bladder capacity (mL) = weight (kg) × 7.
- In child over 1 year of age, bladder capacity (mL) = (age in years + 2) × 30.

A plain X-ray film is taken before contrast is injected. Subsequently, anteroposterior films are taken during filling phase, in full bladder, during micturition and postvoid. Also, the oblique views of bladder and urethra are taken to view the UVJ and urethra, respectively.

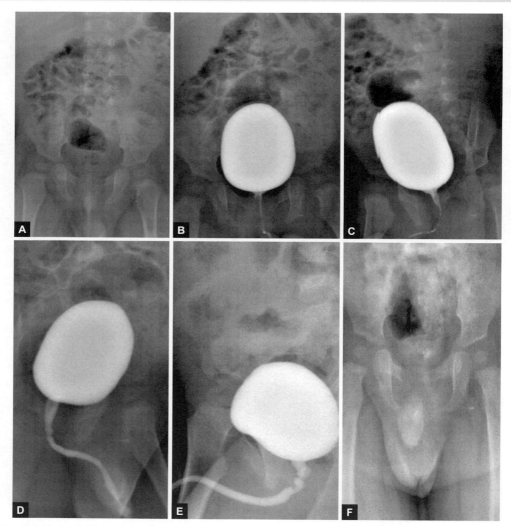

Figs. 6.19A to F: Normal voiding cystourethrogram. (A) Scout film; (B) Full bladder showing normal bladder (frontal view); (C) Full bladder (oblique view); (D) Voiding film showing normal bladder and urethra (frontal view); (E) Voiding film (oblique view); (F) Postvoid film showing no postvoid residue.

Vesicoureteral Reflux

Vesicoureteral reflux is characterized by retrograde flow of urine from bladder to ureter or kidney. It may be an isolated abnormality (primary VUR) or associated with other congenital anomalies of kidney and urinary tract, including renal dysplasia, and obstructive uropathy or neurogenic bladder (secondary VUR).

Grading of VUR

International grading system has classified VUR into five grades (Fig. 6.22) based on the appearance of specific features of the VCUG.

Grade I: Reflux in the nondilated ureter.

Grade II: Reflux in the nondilated ureter, renal pelvis, and calyces (Figs. 6.23A to E).

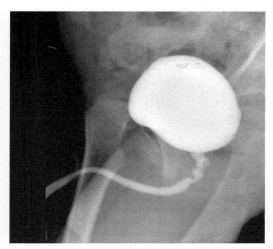

Fig. 6.20: Voiding cystourethrogram showing indentation of the proximal bulbar urethra by the compressor nudae muscle. Normal variant.

Grade III: Mild dilatation of the ureter, renal pelvis, and calyces, with minimal blunting of the fornices.

Grade IV: Moderate ureteral tortuosity and dilatation of renal pelvis and calyces.

Grade V: Gross ureteral dilatation and tortuosity, dilatation of renal pelvis, and calyces and loss of papillary impressions (Figs. 6.24A and B).

Grading of VUR is useful in deciding treatment, follow-up, and predicting outcome of the disease. Lower-grade VURs (Grades I and II) are supposed to resolve spontaneously with age, while higher grade VUR (Grades III, IV, and V) are likely to persist and may need surgery.

Abnormalities of the Urethra

Posterior Urethral Valve

Posterior urethral valve is the most common cause of neonatal lower urinary tract obstruction and the leading cause of end-stage renal disease in males. It results from the abnormal development of a valve-like membrane from the verumontanum to the prostatic urethra. PUV is often suspected in a

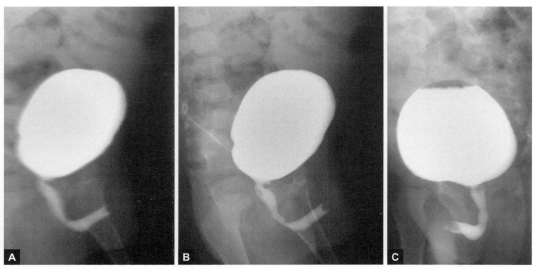

Figs. 6.21A to C: Urethral stone. Voiding cystourethrogram showing filling defect in contrast filled anterior urethra.

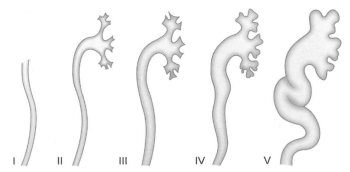

Fig. 6.22: International classification of VUR. Grade I: Reflux into nondilated distal ureter; Grade II: Reflux up to nondilated pelvicalyceal system; Grade III: Reflux into mildly dilated ureter, with minimal blunting of calyceal fornices; Grade IV: Reflux into the moderately dilated ureter and pelvis with blunting of calyceal fornices; Grade V: Reflux into grossly dilated and tortuous ureter with loss of papillary impressions.

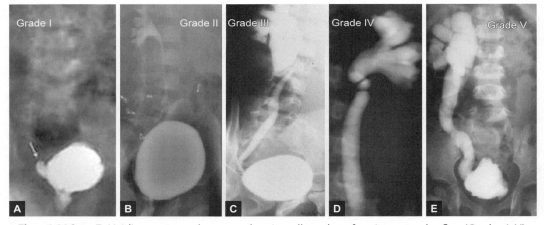

Figs. 6.23A to E: Voiding cystourethrogram showing all grades of vesicoureteral reflux (Grades I–V).

male child with antenatal sonography finding of bilateral hydroureteronephrosis, thick-walled bladder, and diminished amniotic fluid volume. Clinically, it may present as poor urinary stream, acute urinary retention, UTI, or incontinence in a male child. USG is the initial investigation of choice, followed by VCUG. VCUG is considered as gold standard in diagnosis of PUV; showing dilated posterior urethra with abrupt narrowing at the

site of the obstruction, thickened and irregular bladder wall with or without reflux. In severe cases, bladder diverticulum can be seen (Figs. 6.25 and 6.26).

Anterior Urethral Valve and Its Stricture and Diverticulum

Anterior urethral abnormalities are less commonly seen than posterior urethra. VCUG is the investigative modality of choice for

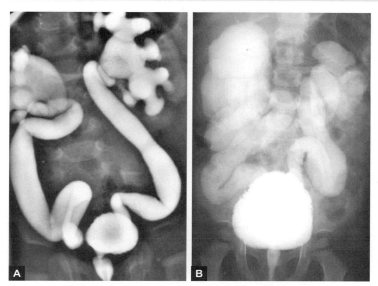

Figs. 6.24A and B: Voiding cystourethrogram showing bilateral Grade V vesicoureteral reflux.

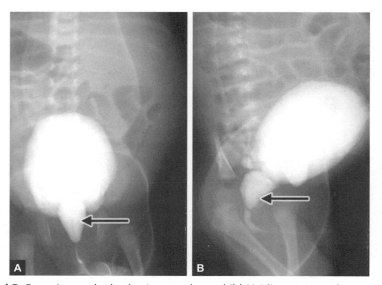

Figs. 6.25A and B: Posterior urethral valve in a newborn child. Voiding cystourethrogram shows dilated and elongated posterior urethra (arrow) and thin stream of contrast in anterior urethra. No vesicoureteric reflux is seen.

anterior urethral valve. It shows dilatation proximal to the valve and narrowing distal to it (Fig. 6.27). Anterior urethral diverticulum is

the second most common cause of congenital urethral obstruction in boys. It is a saccular outpouching of the ventral aspect of the

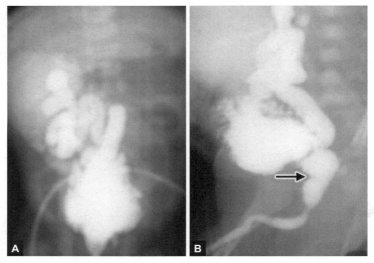

Figs. 6.26A and B: Posterior urethral valve with right-sided Grade V reflux. Bladder shows multiple diverticulae. Posterior urethra is dilated and elongated (arrow).

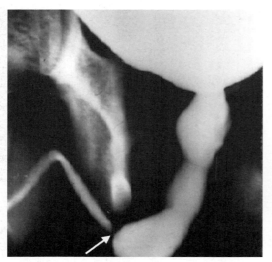

Fig. 6.27: Anterior urethral valve. Voiding cystourethrogram shows urethral dilatation proximal to valve (arrow) and narrowing distal to it.

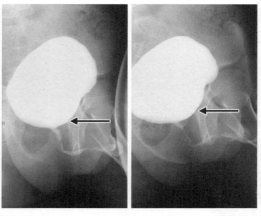

Fig. 6.28: Urethral diverticulum. Voiding cystourethrogram shows a saccular outpouching (arrow) of the proximal part of bulbar urethra.

Abnormalities of the Urinary Bladder

Neurogenic Bladder

anterior urethra near penoscrotal junction. VCUG shows as filling of the diverticulum with the contrast and appears as an oval-shaped structure on the ventral aspect of the anterior urethra (Fig. 6.28).

Spinal dysraphism, sacral malformations, tethered spinal cord, sacrococcygeal teratoma, and spinal cord tumor may result in bladder dysfunction in children. Children may present with urinary incontinence or repeated UTIs. Evaluation of these children starts with complete physical examination to assess the lumbosacral spine for sacral dimples, hairy tufts, hemangiomas, and lipomas. USG of kidney and bladder may show bilateral hydroureteronephrosis and bladder wall thickening with significant postvoid residual urine volume in advanced stages. Children with suspected tethered spinal cord need to be evaluated with MRI spine. VCUG is advised in cases with febrile UTI or upper urinary tract involvement shown by USG. VCUG characteristically shows large and irregular bladder with varying degrees of trabeculation and sacculation with or without reflux (Fig. 6.29). "Christmas tree appearance," elongated upward pointing bladder, may be seen in advanced stages of neurogenic bladder.

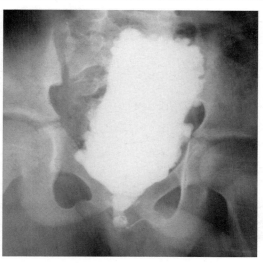

Fig. 6.29: Neurogenic bladder. Voiding cystourethrogram showing large, elongated bladder with trabeculations and sacculations.

Bladder Diverticulae

Bladder diverticulae are localized outpouchings of the bladder mucosa between fibers of the detrusor muscles, resulting from congenital or acquired defect in the bladder wall. A primary bladder diverticulum is usually congenital and most commonly seen in paraureteral region. It can be associated with various syndromes like cutis laxa, Ehlers-Danlos syndrome, etc. A large diverticulum may sometime lead to bladder outlet obstruction (Figs. 6.30A and B). Reflux may be

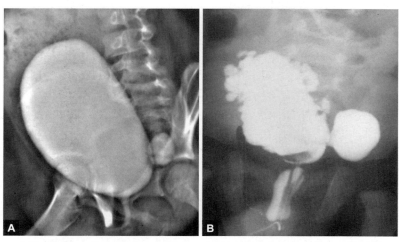

Figs. 6.30A and B: Bladder diverticulum. (A) Simple bladder diverticulum; (B) Bladder diverticulum secondary to bladder outlet obstruction due to posterior urethral valve.

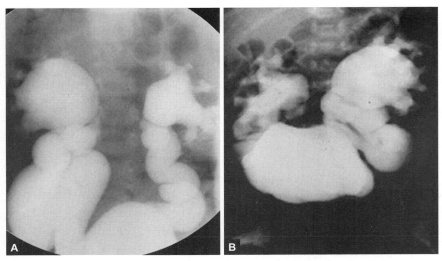

Figs. 6.31A and B: Megacystis-Megaureter. Voiding cystourethrogram showing large capacity bladder with bilateral massively dilated ureter.

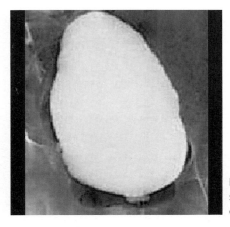

Fig. 6.32: Megacystis. Voiding cystourethrogram showing large capacity bladder in a girl with voiding dysfunction and recurrent urinary tract infections.

associated in half of the cases with bladder diverticulum. Secondary diverticulae are multiple and associated with PUV or neurogenic bladder.

Megacystis

Megacystis is a congenital condition, where bladder is large and smooth-walled, commonly seen in association with refluxing, massively dilated ureters, known as megacystis megaureter syndrome (Figs. 6.31A and B). This condition may be seen in various syndromes like microcolon-intestinal hypoperistalsis syndrome, Ehlers-Danlos syndrome, Prune Belly syndrome, etc.

A large capacity atonic bladder may be seen in female child with voiding dysfunction and recurrent UTI (Fig. 6.32), termed as "lazy bladder syndrome."

Neonatology

Anoop Verma, Kavita Menghani, Pulak Parag

■ NEONATAL CHEST X-RAY

❏ In spite of recent modalities like ultrasound and computerized tomography (CT) scan/magnetic resonance imaging (MRI) conventional radiography is still the cornerstone of imaging.

❏ Film should be technically satisfactory, so that lungs, soft tissue, and bones can be visualized.

❏ The chest should be straight so that both hemithorax in the normal situation would appear the same density.

❏ X-ray should be taken in full inspiration if at all possible.

❏ Mediastinum in a neonate has much variability and consists of mainly heart and thymus. The thymus can fill the whole of the upper mediastinum or is prominent on the right side or the left. In difficult situation especially mass in the mediastinum, ultrasonography remains the investigation of choice. An enlarged thymus has an even texture similar to liver where an abdominal mass will almost certainly have a mixed echogenic pattern.

❏ Apart from viewing pulmonary cardiac and pleural pathology, neonatal X-ray is used to demonstrate the position of various lines and tubes. All those who are dealing with neonatal diseases must be aware of their appearance.

• *Endotracheal tube*: Endotracheal tube (ET) usually has an opaque line in the side of it, making it clearly visible on a plain X-ray. The tip of the tube should lie in between the level of the seventh cervical vertebrae (C7) (just below the larynx) and the level of carina, which is usually around the level of T4 vertebra (Fig. 7.1).

• *Umbilical arterial line*: Umbilical arterial line marked by opaque lines. Position is confirmed by course of catheter which descends into the pelvis to enter the internal iliac artery on either

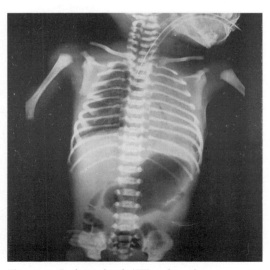

Fig. 7.1: Endotracheal (ET) tube placement: tip should lie between C7 and T4 vertebrae.
Courtesy: Dr. Jagdish Menghani MD, Raipur.

side and then via the common iliac artery into the aorta. The tip of the line should lie between T4 and T10.

- Umbilical venous catheter: Umbilical venous catheter passes through the umbilical vein (uv) and through the liver entering the portal venous system, before passing through the ductus venosus to lie with their tip in the inferior vena cava.

X-ray interpretation: Follow the following steps:

☐ Abdomen: Watch for bowel gas pattern, free intraperitoneal gas, abnormal calcification, abdominal situs, and diaphragmatic position.

☐ Bone: Check for bone density, fracture, lytic and blastic lesion, and features of metabolic bone diseases.

☐ Chest: Look for trachea, mediastinum, cardiac contour, position of aortic arch, pleural effusion, pulmonary vascularity, infiltrates, and atelectasis. In older infants and children, a good inspiratory chest film is one in which the relationship of the sixth anterior rib ends intersect the domes of the diaphragm. This may be difficult to evaluate in neonates where proper positioning is difficult.

Pneumothorax

☐ An area within the chest containing no lung markings with the edge of the lung clearly seen separating from the lungs.

☐ Sometime small pneumothorax, which lies anteriorly, cannot be picked by these signs. There is hypertransradiancy of the chest on the affected side, which can only be identified by high quality film that is not rotated.

The appearance of the heart border or mediastinum appears clearer than in the usual

situation where lung abuts the mediastinum giving the "etched heart border" (Fig. 7.2).

Pneumomediastinum

Also gives the "etched heart border" and is difficult to diagnose with small anterior mediastinum.

Pneumopericardium

Also gives the same sign, but restricted to cardiac contour.

Fluid/Consolidation

Lung opacity, especially if it is uniform poses difficulty in coming to conclusion that one is dealing with fluid or consolidation.

Presence of air bronchogram appearance depicts that opacity is out of the lungs, e.g. consolidation (Fig. 7.3), hyaline membrane disease (HMD), or pulmonary edema.

If the shadow has no particular character, it can be pulmonary edema, infection, hemorrhage, or fluid in the pleural space.

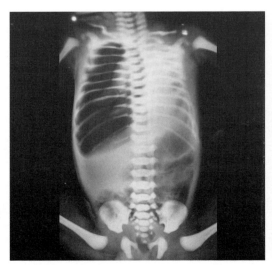

Fig. 7.2: Pneumothorax right. Note the hypertranslucency on left side with mediastinal shift to left side.

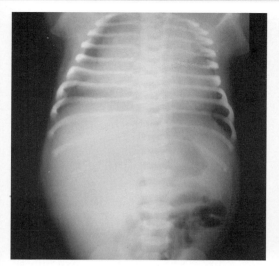

Fig. 7.3: Bilateral lung opacity with air bronchogram indicates the origin is from the lungs suggestive of pneumonia.

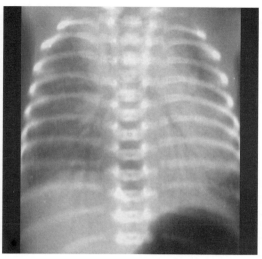

Fig. 7.4: Hyaline membrane disease (chest X-ray) showing granular opacities with air bronchogram.

Normal Neonatal Chest

Prominent Thymus

The thymus is a thin, bilobed organ located in the superior mediastinum that has a variable size and shape. The thymus lies anteriorly in relationship to the heart and great vessels.

The relative size of the thymus increases with expiration and decreases with inspiration.

The thymus decreases in size during periods of stress, such as during sepsis. Because the thymus is a soft organ, overlying ribs may indent it, causing a "wave" sign. The right lobe of the thymus can insinuate into the minor fissure, causing a "sail" sign.

Hyaline Membrane Disease

General Considerations

❑ Lack of sufficient surfactant production inadequate pressure to keep alveoli open, which decreases the lung compliance.

❑ Neonates predisposed are premature infants under 34 weeks, babies delivered out of cesarean section and infants of diabetic mothers.

❑ Neonates are prone to respiratory distress syndrome.

❑ Surfactant therapy changes the radiographic picture of HMD.

X-ray Appearance

❑ Typically, diffuse "ground-glass" or finely granular appearance, which is bilateral and symmetrical in distribution (Fig. 7.4).

❑ Presence of air bronchogram especially extending peripherally.

❑ Hypoaeration in nonventilated lung and hyperinflation excludes HMD.

Transient Tachypnea of the Newborn

General Considerations

❑ Transient tachypnea of the newborn (TTN), also called retained fetal lung fluid or "wet lung", is a diagnosis of exclusion.

- Usually full-term or slightly preterm delivered by cesarean section and some by precipitous labor.
- Mild respiratory distress immediately after birth.
- Improve within several hours.
- Because the symptoms and radiological features are nonspecific, infection should be considered in the differential diagnosis. Typically, respiratory symptoms resolve within the first 24 hours of life, but occasionally can persist longer.

X-ray Appearance

- Hyperinflation of the lungs (Fig. 7.5)
- Strand-like opacities originating from hilum
- Fluid in the fissures
- Laminar effusions
- Strand like opacities through the vessels
- Cardiomegaly.

Meconium Aspiration Syndrome

General Considerations

This is the most common cause of neonatal respiratory distress in full-term/postmature infants.

Imaging Findings

- Diffuse "ropey" densities (similar to bronchopulmonary dysplasia). These heterogeneous opacities are seen in central two-thirds of the lung.
- There are patchy areas of atelectasis and emphysema from air trapping.
- Hyperinflation of lungs and spontaneous pneumothorax and pneumomediastinum (Fig. 7.6).

Pulmonary Hypoplasia

- Lung growth depends on adequacy of amniotic fluid and obviously in oligohydramnios there is hypoplasia of both lungs (Potter syndrome).

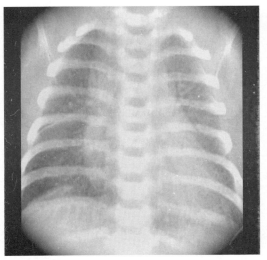

Fig. 7.5: Transient tachypnea of the newborn: X-ray of newborn with respiratory distress soon after birth, note hyperinflation of lungs and strands of opacities coming out of hilum.

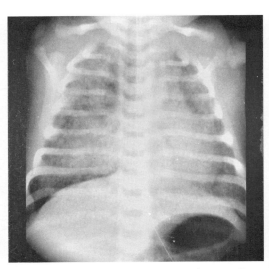

Fig. 7.6: Meconium aspiration syndrome: Chest X-ray reveals bilateral patchy opacities with pocket of hyperinflation.

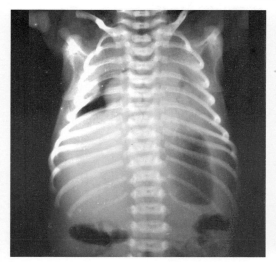

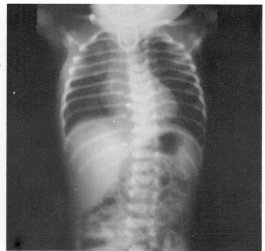

Fig. 7.7: Pulmonary hypoplasia. Narrow chest with distended abdomen and a small pocket of pneumothorax representing friable lungs. A case of potter syndrome clinically.

Fig. 7.8: Esophageal atresia. Note the coiling of the infant feeding tube at upper esophageal pouch.

- Lungs are friable and easily ruptured giving rise to pneumothorax.
- Unilateral hypoplasia is a feature of diaphragmatic hernia.
- Lung hypoplasia is best defined as the ratio of lung weight to body weight—clearly a pathological diagnosis.
- Hypoplasia of the lungs is difficult to detect by X-ray. In a case of unexplained pneumothorax, renal ultrasonography (USG) will give valuable information (Fig. 7.7) as in Potter syndrome.

Esophageal Atresia

Esophageal atresia is the most common congenital abnormality of esophagus, and is associated with 50–70% chance of other congenital abnormalities.

Types

- Seventy percent of the esophageal atresia with distal tracheoesophageal fistula

- In 10–15%, there is no fistula between atretic esophagus and trachea, the two esophagus segments are separated widely.
- In 5%, there is no atresia, but an "H-type" communication exists between the trachea and the esophagus.
- Rest two other types are very rare where isolated fistula of superior segment and fistula of both upper and lower segment of an atretic esophagus are present.
- Chest X-ray reveals lucency over the cervical and upper thoracic spine due to blind ending pouch of esophagus is filled with air (Fig. 7.8).
- Lateral chest view showing the blind esophagus pouch and the anterior bowing and narrowing of the trachea.
- A complete gasless abdomen is the hallmark of esophageal atresia without fistula.
- Fluoroscopic examination with barium helps in presurgical evaluation.
- The tip of the arrested catheter in the air-filled pouch may offer similar information.
- Diagnosis of H-type of fistula may be difficult.

Congenital Diaphragmatic Hernia

- ❑ Incidence of congenital diaphragmatic hernia is 1 in 2,000 to 1 in 5,000 live births.
- ❑ It is associated with stillbirths, anomalies of chorionic villus sampling (CVS), gastrointestinal tract (GIT), vertebral, genitourinary, neural tube development, and chromosomal anomalies like trisomies 13, 13, 21.
- ❑ Diaphragmatic hernia is a syndrome where hernia is accompanied by pulmonary hypoplasia, lung immaturity, and left heart hypoplasia leading to persistent pulmonary hypertension of the newborn. There are three types of congenital diaphragmatic hernia.

Clinical Features

Neonate presents with acute respiratory distress with a scaphoid abdomen. Bowel sounds are audible on the herniated hemithorax. Plain X-ray chest and abdomen shows, mediastinal shift to opposite side. The ipsilateral hemithorax contains bowel loops filled with gas. There is paucity of intestinal loops in the abdomen (Figs. 7.9 and 7.10). The ipsilateral lung is hypoplastic. Herniation of stomach into the thorax is not necessary be always there in congenital diaphragmatic hernia.

Differential Diagnosis

Congenital diaphragmatic hernia has to be differentiated from eventration of diaphragm and congenital cystic adenomatoid malformation.

Eventration of Diaphragm

Eventration (e out + venter belly or "out of belly") is an abnormal elevation of one, or part of one, intact leaf of the diaphragm and it differs from a diaphragmatic hernia in that there is defect in the later.

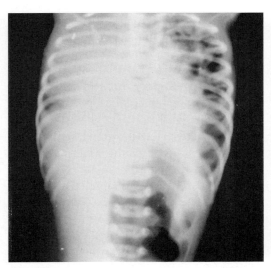

Fig. 7.9: Congenital diaphragmatic hernia. Intestine loops are visible at left hemithorax with shift of mediastinum to right side.

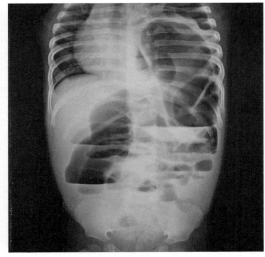

Fig. 7.10: Congenital diaphragmatic hernia with intestinal obstruction: A Meckel's band causing small intestinal obstruction.

Etiology

Eventration of diaphragm is either congenital or acquired.

Acquired: Paralysis of phrenic nerve.

Congenital: Sac of eventration is difficult to differentiate from a diaphragmatic hernia.

Clinical Features

Ranges from totally asymptomatic infant to wheezing, respiratory infections, and exercise intolerance.

Diagnosis

❑ Presence of elevation of diaphragm contour. In severe cases, the eventration may actually cause symptom as does the hernia, like shift of mediastinum to opposite side, hypoplasia of ipsilateral lung (Fig. 7.11). Occasionally eventration may allow liver (Fig. 7.12), kidney, or rarely spleen to assume intrathoracic position.

❑ In fluoroscopy of the chest, the diaphragm moves paradoxically with respiratory motion.

❑ Computerized tomography scan and MRI are used now frequently to make the diagnosis.

Examination of Abdomen

❑ There are three common X-ray densities on a plain X-ray abdomen soft tissue/fluid, gas, and calcification.

❑ Calcification within the peritoneum is seen in meconium peritonitis.

❑ Intraluminal colonic calcification is seen in bowel/urinary tract communication.

Common queries in plain X-ray abdomen.

Which type of bowel is it?

The large bowel appears round toward periphery of the abdomen; otherwise it is difficult to distinguish between the two (Fig. 7.13).

Presence of Free Air

❑ There is diffuse radiolucency over the upper abdomen toward liver.

❑ Both sides of the bowel wall are visualized.

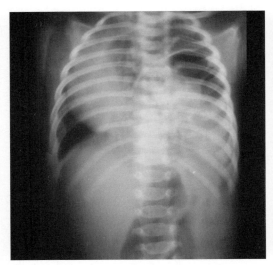

Fig. 7.11: Eventration of diaphragm left. Note the shift of mediastinum.

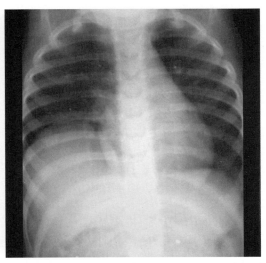

Fig. 7.12: Eventration of diaphragm. Liver found inside the right chest.

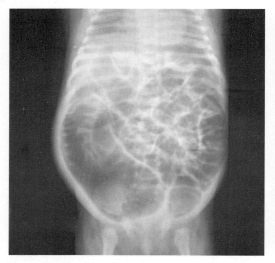

Fig. 7.13: The large bowel seen toward periphery of the abdomen.

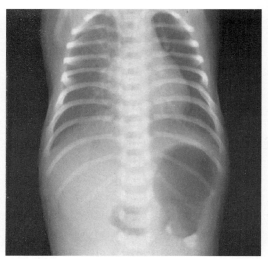

Fig. 7.14: Duodenal stenosis. A plain X-ray of a baby presenting with bilious vomiting and abdominal distension—the double bubble sign.

❏ *Presence of free fluid*: Since there is scanty, bowel gas in neonate free fluid is difficult to pick up by plain X-ray, but if the bowel loops remains centrally in the abdomen it gives clue to the presence of free fluid. Ultrasonography is better in detecting free fluid in the abdomen.

❏ *Presence of necrotizing entercolitis*: The presence of gas in the bowel wall as linear streaks or curvilinear pattern and appears like bubbles. Fixed bowel loops pattern from one to another radiograph.

❏ *Presence of ileus or obstruction*: If the dilatation of bowel is uniform, it favors ileus and if there is more dilatation of distal than proximal then obstruction is more likely the diagnosis.

Duodenal Atresias and Stenosis

❏ Duodenal atresia results from failure of recanalization. Most of atresia involve second and third part of the duodenum and are located distal to the common bile duct.

❏ Incomplete recanalization can lead to duodenal stenosis or the presence of duodenal bulb. The extrinsic causes of partial obstruction are due to annular pancreas, presence of Ladd's band.

❏ Association of polyhydramnios, trisomy 21, vertebral defects, cardiac, and renal anomalies are there.

Diagnosis

Presence of "double bubble sign" represents simultaneous distension of stomach and the first part of the duodenum (Figs. 7.14 and 7.15). This appearance is highlighted if the stomach is aspirated via nasogastric tube and 50 mL of air is instilled. This is the isolated finding in one-third to one-half of cases.

Ileal Atresia

❏ Atresia of jejunum and ileum is often caused by interruption of blood supply to fetal gut.

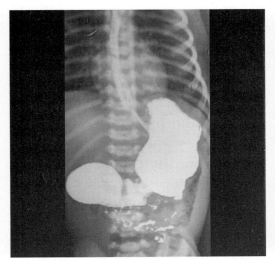

Fig. 7.15: Duodenal atresia: Barium study.

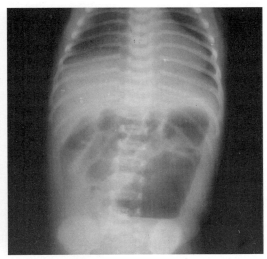

Fig. 7.16: Ileal atresia. Plain X-ray abdomen showing distended bowel loop with fluid level.

❏ Jejunoileal atresia is classified into four types:
1. *Type I*: Membranous atresia with intact bowel wall and mesentery
2. *Type II*: Two atretic blind ends connected by a fibrous cord with an intact mesentery
3. *Type IIIA*: Two ends of the atretic bowel separated by V-shaped mesenteric defect. It is the most common and is associated with short bowel length. *Type IIIB*: This is called as apple peel deformity and consists of proximal jejunal atresia, a wide mesenteric gap, and a distal small bowel segment coiled around a marginal artery.
4. *Type IV*: Multiple atresia (sting of sausages).

Plain X-ray Abdomen

❏ Demonstrate picture of intestinal obstruction and multiple fluid level (Fig. 7.16). The more the distal obstruction greater are the number of distended bowel.
❏ Bowel may perforate and meconium can enter into the peritoneal cavity and

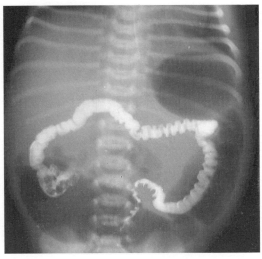

Fig. 7.17: Ileal atresia. Contrast enema reveals the unused microcolon.
Courtesy: Dr. Pulak Parag, MCh, Raipur.

calcify. It is a fact that normal meconium is more likely to calcify in the peritoneum rather than abnormal meconium of cystic fibrosis. Contrast enema gives a picture of unused microcolon (Fig. 7.17).

Colonic Atresia

Colonic atresia is less common than ileal atresia. It has to be differentiated from obstruction of distal ileum because plain X-ray suggests a low intestinal obstruction.

The proximal portion to atresia or obstruction is grossly dilated and mottles pattern of gas can be seen and meconium can be visualized (Fig. 7.18). Contrast enema depicts the presence of microcolon with inability to enter the proximal dilated colon (Fig. 7.19).

Malrotation with Paraduodenal Hernia

Malrotation of the small intestine may present as intestinal obstruction (Fig. 7.20).

Meconium Peritonitis

❑ Meconium ileus is caused by obstruction of small intestine by highly viscid meconium. About 15% cases are associated with cystic fibrosis.

❑ It is of two types, uncomplicated or complicated. In uncomplicated, the obstruction is at small terminal bowel as a result proximal bowel is dilated and distal colon is unused or turns to microcolon. In complicated, there is volvulus of meconium-laden pellets in the fetus, which may result into perforation, peritonitis, and meconium pseudocyst formation or ileal atresia.

❑ Neonate presents with palpable intestinal loops and here may be palpable

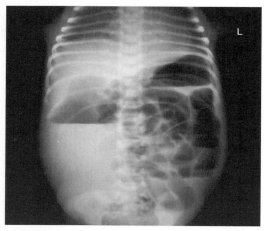

Fig. 7.18: Colonic atresia. Note the grossly dilated bowel shadow.

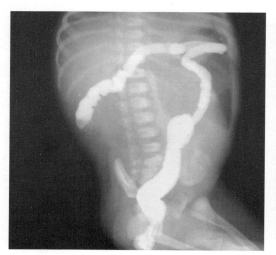

Fig. 7.19: Contrast enema depicts the presence of microcolon.

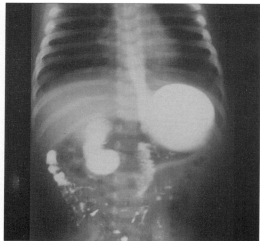

Fig. 7.20: Malrotation with paraduodenal hernia.

abdominal mass. Delay in passage of meconium, or passage of meconium pellets.

- Plain X-ray of abdomen depicts marked bowel distension, soap bubble appearance caused by admixture of air and viscid meconium (Fig. 7.21). In complicated cases, intraperitoneal calcification and pseudocyst formation is seen (Fig. 7.22). Contrast isotonic enema is diagnostic and reveals unused microcolon. Complicated cases require operation.

Hirschsprung's Disease

- Hirschsprung's disease is characterized by congenital absence of intramural ganglionic cells in the rectum.
- *Short segment Hirschsprung's disease*: The aganglionosis is restricted to the rectum and sigmoid colon in 75% of patients.
- *Large segment Hirschsprung's disease*: The aganglionosis extends to splenic flexure or transverse colon and is seen in 15% of patients.
- *Total colonic aganglionosis*: The aganglionosis extends to cover whole colon and variable length of terminal ileum in 8% of cases.

Inheritance

Sporadic mostly, but autosomal dominant, autosomal recessive and polygenic pattern of inheritance is seen. Association with Down's syndrome, Waardenburg syndrome is known. Cardiac, genitourinary, nervous system, and gastrointestinal system defects are recorded in 5% cases of Hirschsprung's disease.

Clinical Features

- Delayed passage of meconium beyond 48 hours in full-term baby is pathognomic of Hirschsprung's disease. Abdominal distension and feed refusal vomiting are other association in this disease.

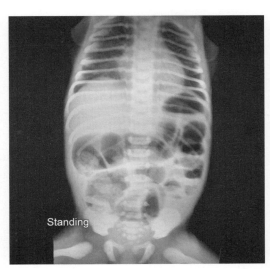

Fig. 7.21: Meconium ileus: a baby presenting with intestinal obstruction showing absence of air-fluid levels and soap bubble appearance in the right lower abdomen.

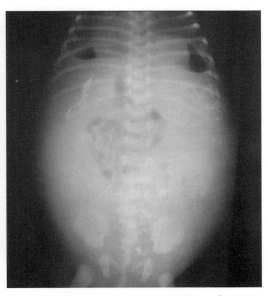

Fig. 7.22: Meconium peritonitis: X-ray depicting hazy abdomen with intraperitoneal calcification.

- Rectal examination again gives you important clue. There is tight contracted anorectal junction and withdraw of the finger may be followed by explosive discharge of stool and gas.
- Plain X-ray of abdomen reveals multiple dilated loops of bowel with an absent rectal gas shadow (see Fig. 7.13).
- Contrast enema performed by isotonic water-soluble contrast media gives typically a narrow distal segment of rectum, a cone-shaped transition zone, and a proximal dilated colon (Fig. 7.23). Anorectal manometry is not performed nowadays. Rectal biopsy is taken usually from 2 to 4 cm from the anal verge. Diagnosis will depend on absence of ganglionic cell, thickened nerve trunks, and a marked increase in acetylcholinesterase activity in the hypertrophied nerve bundle.

Necrotizing Enterocolitis

- Necrotizing enterocolitis is a serious gastrointestinal disease of neonates. Its etiology is unknown. Necrotizing enterocolitis is characterized by mucosal or transmucosal necrosis of part of the intestine. Infants born before term who are undersized and ill are most susceptible to necrotizing enterocolitis.
- Abdominal radiographs may demonstrate multiple dilated bowel loops that display little or no change in location and appearance with sequential studies. Pneumatosis intestinalis gas in the bowel wall (Fig. 7.24) that displays a linear or bubbly pattern is present in 50–75% of patients. Ultrasonography of the abdomen characteristically shows thick-walled loops of bowel with hypomotility. Intraperitoneal fluid is often present. In the presence of pneumatosis intestinalis,

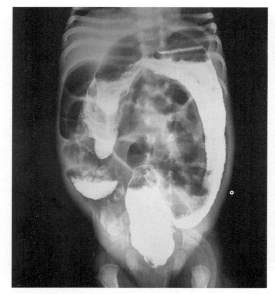

Fig. 7.23: Hirschsprung's disease: Barium enema depicting dilated segment of proximal colon. *Courtesy:* Dr. Pulak Parag, MCh, Raipur.

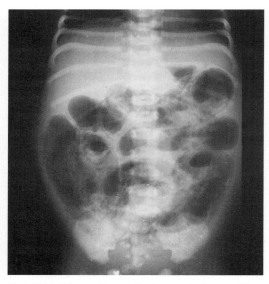

Fig. 7.24: The radiograph demonstrates multiple dilated loops in the large bowel and small bowel. Note the pneumatosis intestinalis with bubbly and linear gas collections in the bowel wall.

gas is seen in the portal venous circulation within the liver.

Pneumoperitoneum

❑ Neonatal pneumoperitoneum remains a surgical emergency and outcome can be lethal if the problem is not addressed early. It is an alarming Roentgen sign in the overwhelming majority of cases indicative of perforation of the GIT, for which immediate laparotomy is indicated.

❑ *Causes*: Necrotizing enterocolitis remained the single major cause of pneumoperitoneum in the newborn; however, in 44 (49.4%) patients the cause was not related to necrotizing enterocolitis. Perforated pouch colon, isolated colonic perforations, caecal perforations, gastric, and duodenal perforations were the main causes of pneumoperitoneum not related to necrotizing enterocolitis.

❑ In a small number of cases, intraperitoneal air has been described to occur with pneumomediastinum and/or pneumothorax. It is thought that air dissects from the mediastinum into the retroperitoneal tissues through the diaphragmatic foramina and then descends between the leaves of the mesentery with final rupture into the free peritoneal space. The clue to the benign nature of free intraperitoneal air in these cases is the simultaneous radiographic evidence of pneumomediastinum and/or pneumothorax.

❑ Football sign, which is seen on supine abdominal radiographs, refers to a large oval radiolucency in the shape of an American football. The long axis of the "football" runs cephalocaudad, and the blunted ends are defined by the diaphragm and pelvic floor. A well-defined and vertically oriented linear opacity may

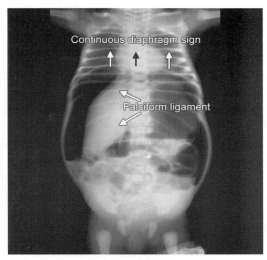

Fig. 7.25: Pneumoperitoneum: This is huge collection of gas under diaphragm. There is continuous diaphragm sign and falciform ligament is easily seen.

be identified within the cephalic portion of the radiolucency, overlying the right upper abdomen. An additional, well-defined and vertically oriented linear opacity may be seen within the caudal portion of the radiolucency, overlying the midline of the lower abdomen.

❑ *Continuous diaphragm sign*: There is of air across the spine simulating a complete diaphragm from side to side (Fig. 7.25).

Gastroesophageal Reflux

❑ It refers to immaturity of lower esophageal sphincter function, manifested by frequent transient lower esophageal relaxations that results in retrograde flow of gastric contents into the esophagus.

❑ As many as 60–70% of infants experience emesis during at least one feeding per 24 hour period by age 3–4 months. The distinction between this "physiologic" gastroesophageal reflux and "pathologic" gastroesophageal reflux in infancy and childhood is determined, not merely by the number and severity of reflux episodes (when assessed by intraesophageal pH monitoring), but is most importantly determined by the presence of reflux-related complications, including failure to thrive, erosive esophagitis, esophageal stricture formation, and chronic respiratory disease.

❐ Gastroesophageal reflux is classified as follows:
  • *Physiologic (or functional) gastroesophageal reflux*: These patients have no underlying predisposing factors or conditions. Growth and development are normal, and pharmacologic treatment is typically not necessary.
  • *Pathologic gastroesophageal reflux or gastroesophageal reflux disease*: Patients frequently experience complications noted above, requiring careful evaluation and treatment.
  • *Secondary gastroesophageal reflux*: This refers to a case in which an underlying condition may predispose to gastroesophageal reflux. Examples include asthma (a condition that may also be, in part, caused by or exacerbated by reflux) and gastric outlet obstruction.

❐ Upper GI imaging series
  This is used to evaluate the anatomy of the upper GI tract, but contrast imaging

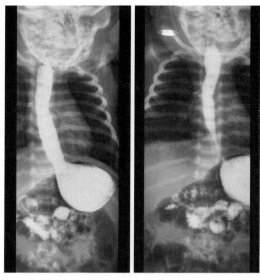

Fig. 7.26: Gastroesophageal reflux: barium study reveals reflux of barium back to esophagus. *Courtesy*: Kavita Menghani, Raipur.

studies are neither sensitive nor specific for gastroesophageal reflux.

Imaging may be useful in the evaluation of gastric emptying time, which may be delayed in gastroesophageal reflux.

Gastric scintiscan: This imaging study, using milk or formula that contains a small amount of technetium sulfur colloid, can assess gastric emptying and can reveal reflux (Fig. 7.26). However, its major diagnostic role is in the assessment of pulmonary aspiration.

Interesting Case Scenarios

TM Ananda Kesavan, TU Sukumaran

■ INTERESTING RESPIRATORY CASES

Case 1 (Figs. 8.1 and 8.2)

❑ A 9-year-old boy presented with fever and cough of 7 days duration and facial puffiness

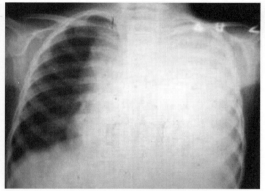

Fig. 8.1: Radiograph showing opacity on left side and irregular right cardiac border. Left costophrenic angle not obliterated.

❑ Radiograph showing opacity on left side (left costophrenic angle is not obliterated) and irregular right cardiac border
❑ Bone marrow proved it as case of non-Hodgkin's lymphoma and chemotherapy was given
❑ Postchemotherapy radiograph showing massive reduction of mass
❑ Beware of tumor lysis syndrome while treating such a large mediastinal mass.

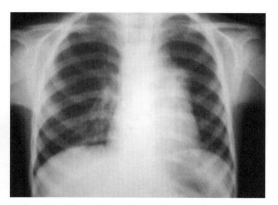

Fig. 8.2: X-ray after chemotherapy for a week.

Case 2 (Figs. 8.3 and 8.4)

❑ A 4-year-old female child presented with "recurrent respiratory tract infection." She had taken several course of antibiotics

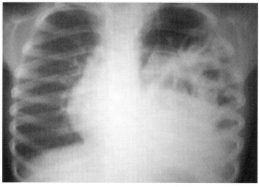

Fig. 8.3: Radiograph showing nonhomogeneous opacity on left side with mediastinal shift.

❏ Radiograph showing nonhomogeneous opacity on left side with mediastinal shift
❏ Diagnosed as a case of diaphragmatic hernia and surgically corrected
❏ Surgically corrected diaphragmatic hernia (intercostal drainage tube in situ)

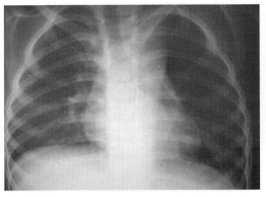

Fig. 8.4: Same child in Figure 8.3 after surgery (intercostal drainage tube in situ).

❏ Diaphragmatic hernia can present at a later age also.

Case 3 (Fig. 8.5)

❏ A case of diaphragmatic hernia presented at 2 years of age

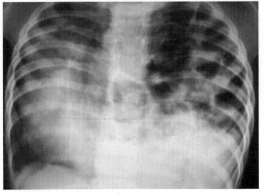

Fig. 8.5: Diaphragmatic hernia.

❏ During surgery, liver and spleen were also there inside the thorax.

Case 4 (Fig. 8.6)

❏ Right-sided diaphragmatic hernia; 90% of diaphragmatic hernias are on left side.

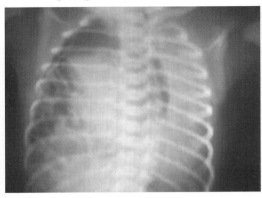

Fig. 8.6: Diaphragmatic hernia on right side.

Case 5 (Fig. 8.7)

❏ A 9-month-old male child admitted with severe respiratory distress and features of cardiac failure. Child was severely anemic and had huge hepatosplenomegaly

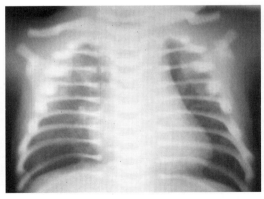

Fig. 8.7: Increased bone density of clavicle and ribs: a case of osteopetrosis.

❏ Radiograph showing increased bone density
❏ Cardiac and lung shadows are normal
❏ X-ray of other bones also showed increased bone density and is diagnostic of osteopetrosis.

Case 6 (Fig. 8.8)

❏ A 7-year-old boy with very severe pneumonia. Child was very toxic

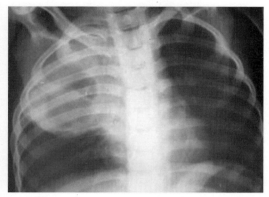

Fig. 8.8: Right upper lobe pneumonia. Note the characteristic bulging of fissure.

❏ Radiograph showing right upper lobe pneumonia with characteristic bulging of fissure
❏ Culture proves it as a case of Klebsiella pneumonia.

Case 7 (Fig. 8.9)

❏ An 11-year-old girl otherwise healthy presented with on and off fever of 1 month duration
❏ X-ray showing miliary tuberculosis.

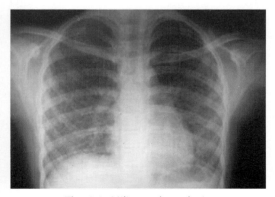

Fig. 8.9: Miliary tuberculosis.

Radiographic Findings in Pulmonary Tuberculosis

❏ No characteristic X-ray finding for pulmonary tuberculosis
❏ Enlarged lymph nodes
❏ Hilar, paratracheal, and subcarinal lymph nodes
❏ Pneumonia and bronchopneumonia
❏ Unilateral pleural effusion
❏ Cavitation is unusual. Suspect when pneumonia not responding to proper antibiotics.

Differential Diagnosis of Miliary Mottling

Suspect when pneumonia not responding to proper antibiotics.
❏ Miliary tuberculosis
❏ Bronchopneumonia: Viral, bacterial, and fungal
❏ Pulmonary edema
❏ Pulmonary infarction
❏ Interstitial lung disease
❏ Hyaline membrane disease (HMD)
❏ Tropical eosinophilia
❏ Aspiration pneumonia
❏ Histiocytosis
❏ Pneumoconiosis
❏ Hemosiderosis.

Case 8 (Figs. 8.10 to 8.13)

❏ A 9-year-old girl with severe pneumonia and not responding to first-line antibiotics
❏ Culture proves it as a case of staphylococcal pneumonia
❏ X-ray showing cavitation, later multiple fluid level. This child also had deep vein thrombosis of right thigh

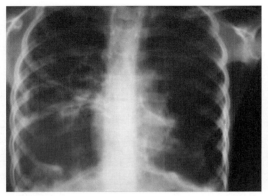

Fig. 8.10: Multiple pneumatocele—suggestive of staphylococcal pneumonia.

❑ Multiple pneumatocele—suggestive of staphylococcal pneumonia

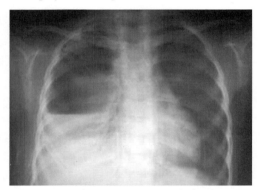

Fig. 8.11: Multiple abscesses with fluid inside.

❑ Radiograph showing multiple fluid level and partially collapsed lung on right side

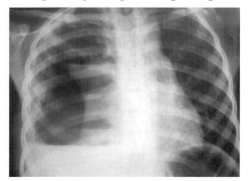

Fig. 8.12: Pneumothorax with partially collapsed lung on right side.

❑ Intercostal drainage tube in situ and also note surgical emphysema.

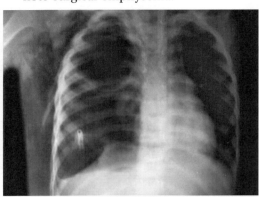

Fig. 8.13: Large pneumatocele with surgical emphysema (Intercostal drainage tube *in situ*).

Case 9 (Fig. 8.14)

❑ A 6-year-old child with recurrent respiratory tract infection since birth

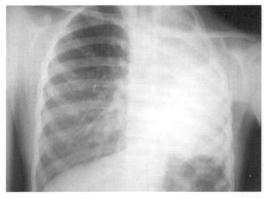

Fig. 8.14: Uniform density on left side with hyperinflated right lung: hypoplastic left lung.

❑ X-ray showing uniform density on left side with hyperinflated right lung
❑ It was a case of hypoplastic left lung and was removed surgically.

Case 10 (Fig. 8.15)

❑ A child with severe pneumonia and respiratory distress.

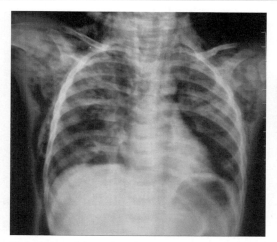

Fig. 8.15: Bilateral subcutaneous emphysema (with pneumonia)

Case 11 (Fig. 8.16)

❑ A 5-year-old child with high-grade fever and features suggestive of severe pneumonia

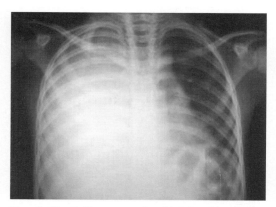

Fig. 8.16: Uniform opacity (right) without any mediastinal shift: uncomplicated pneumonia.

❑ Uniform opacity on right side without any mediastinal shift
❑ Completely resolved after a course of antibiotics
❑ Pneumonia without complications. Note that there is no mediastinal shift and costophrenic angle is free of fluid.

Case 12 (Fig. 8.17)

❑ An 8-year-old child with fever, cough, and breathlessness

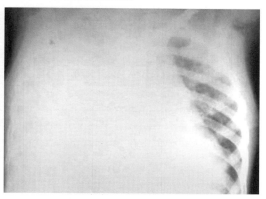

Fig. 8.17: Uniform opacity with mediastinal shift: a case of tuberculosis pleural effusion.

❑ Uniform opacity with mediastinal shift
❑ Pleural fluid was aspirated and diagnosed as a case of tuberculosis.

Case 13 (Fig. 8.18)

❑ A child with complicated pneumonia

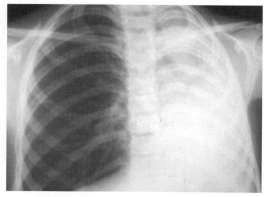

Fig. 8.18: Uniform opacity on left with grossly shifted mediastinum: collapse consolidation.

❑ Uniform opacity on left with grossly shifted trachea. A case of collapse consolidation.

Case numbers 11 to 13 showing uniform opacity on one side of lung.

Differential Diagnosis of Unilateral Lung Opacity

❏ Pleural effusion
❏ Pneumonia
❏ Agenesis
❏ Pneumonectomy
❏ Collapse
❏ Mass lesion.

Case 14 (Fig. 8.19)

❏ A child with cyanotic congenital heart disease with culture-proven infective endocarditis, not responding to multiple antibiotics

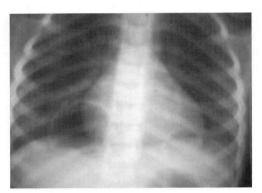

Fig. 8.19: X-ray showing two lung abscesses.

❏ X-ray showing two abscesses.

Case 15 (Fig. 8.20)

❏ A 6-month-old child with fever and cough
❏ Radiograph showing thymic shadow.

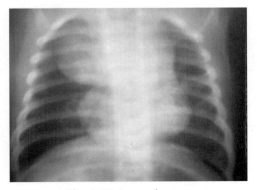

Fig. 8.20: Large thymus.

Differential Diagnosis of Mediastinal Mass

❏ Anterior mediastinum—3Ts: Thyroid, thymus, and teratoma
❏ Posterior mediastinum—3Ns: Neuroblastoma, neurofibroma, and neural crest tumor
❏ Middle mediastinum: Lymph node, pericardial cyst, and bronchial cyst.

Case 16 (Fig. 8.21)

❏ A child with acute respiratory distress

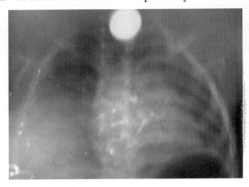

Fig. 8.21: Foreign body (coin) in the larynx.

❏ Importance of asking history of aspiration of food or foreign body. Coin successfully removed.

Case 17 (Fig. 8.22)

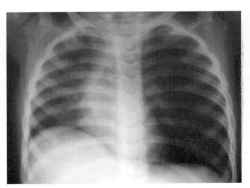

Fig. 8.22: X-ray showing hyperinflation on left side and mediastinal shift to right: foreign body on left bronchus.

- Cough of 7 days duration
- H/o aspiration of ground nut 1 week back
- Air entry decreased on left side
- X-ray showing hyperinflation on left side air trapping and mediastinal shift to right
- Foreign body removed bronchoscopically.

Case 18 (Fig. 8.23)

- Sudden onset of breathlessness.

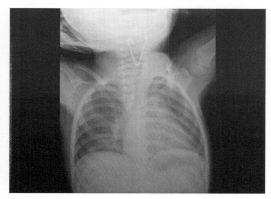

Fig. 8.23: Foreign body (safety pin) in throat

Case 19 (Fig. 8.24)

- Otherwise normal child

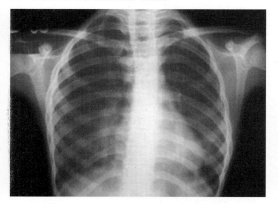

Fig. 8.24: Cervical rib on right side.

- Radiograph showing cervical rib on right side
- Importance of looking outside the lung shadow cannot be overemphasized.

Case 20 (Fig. 8.25)

- A 7-year-old boy with cough and nontoxic

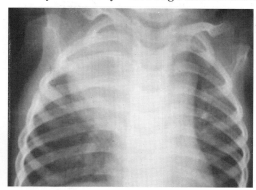

Fig. 8.25: Uniform opacity of right upper part not corresponding to upper lobe zone.

- Was treated with two courses of antibiotics
- Radiograph showing uniform opacity of right upper lobe zone. The shadow is not corresponding anatomically to the upper lobe zone
- Shadow not cleared with a course of antibiotic also
- Child was operated and biopsy proved it as ganglioneuroblastoma
- All white shadows need not be pneumonia.

Case 21 (Fig. 8.26)

- An asymptomatic child.

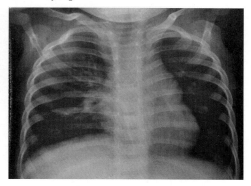

Fig. 8.26: Right-sided cervical rib

Case 22 (Figs. 8.27 and 8.28)

❏ History of recurrent cough and fever

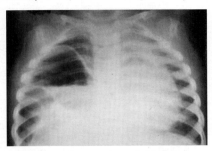

Fig. 8.27: Eventration of diaphragm.

❏ Eventration of diaphragm (right)

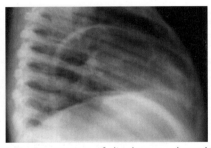

Fig. 8.28: Eventration of diaphragm—lateral view showing elevated dome of right diaphragm.

❏ Lateral view showing elevated dome of right diaphragm.

Case 23 (Figs. 8.29 and 8.30)

❏ An 11-year-old girl
❏ History of recurrent respiratory tract infection
❏ Father and mother died of pneumonia

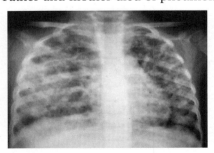

Fig. 8.29: X-ray: bilateral interstitial pneumonia in a child with HIV infection.

❏ X-ray: Bilateral interstitial pneumonia
❏ The child was suffering from AIDS and pneumonia promptly responded to cotri-moxazole (*Pneumocystis jiroveci*)
❏ The child was readmitted after 2 weeks.

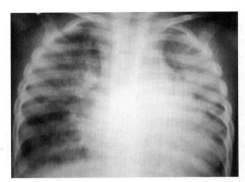

Fig. 8.30: Same child (Fig. 8.29) with large fluffy shadow bilaterally: lymphoid interstitial pneumonia.

❏ Bilateral interstitial pneumonia with large fluffy shadow
❏ Responded to antibiotics and a course of steroid
❏ Probably a case of lymphoid interstitial pneumonia.

Case 24 (Fig. 8.31)

❏ Child with on and off fever and cough

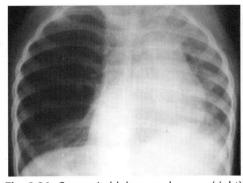

Fig. 8.31: Congenital lobar emphysema (right).

❏ Congenital lobar emphysema.

Case 25 (Fig. 8.32)

❑ Otherwise normal child, general examination showed flattening of left chest

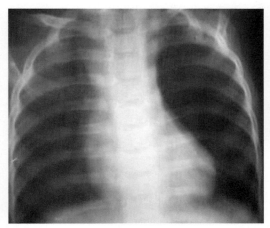

Fig. 8.32: Increased radiolucency (left): Poland syndrome.

❑ Radiograph showing increased radiolucency on left side. It was a case of Poland syndrome.

Differential Diagnosis of Increased Radiolucency on One Side

❑ Pneumothorax
❑ Obstruction due to foreign body
❑ Large bullae
❑ Compensatory emphysema
❑ Mastectomy
❑ Poland syndrome.

Case 26 (Figs. 8.33 and 8.34)

❑ Sudden onset of cough and dyspnea
❑ History of foreign body could not be elicited
❑ Chest X-ray posteroanterior view was normal, and foreign body was detected in lateral view

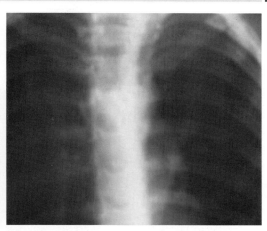

Fig. 8.33: A child with history of foreign body aspiration: chest X-ray posteroanterior view was normal.

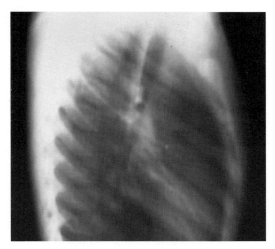

Fig. 8.34: Same child in Figure 8.33—lateral view showing foreign body in the trachea.

❑ Foreign body in the trachea clearly visible in the lateral X-ray, but not seen in posteroanterior view.

Case 27 (Fig. 8.35)

❑ A child with nephrotic syndrome and massive edema.

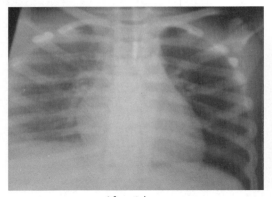

After 1 hour

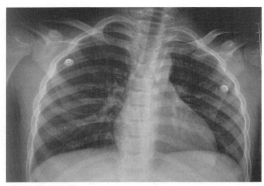

Fig. 8.35: First X-ray was taken when the patient was in right lateral position for long time. After 1 hour right-sided fluid (and shadow) disappeared.

Case 28 (Figs. 8.36 and 8.37)

❏ A preterm newborn with respiratory distress

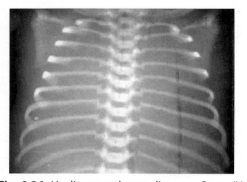

Fig. 8.36: Hyaline membrane disease—Stage IV.

❏ X-ray showing features of HMD—Stage IV

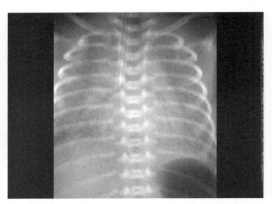

Fig. 8.37: Hyaline membrane disease (HMD) in stage III: heart border just visible.

❏ Radiograph showing HMD stage III: Heart border just visible.

HMD—Staging

❏ Stage I—Mottling
❏ Stage II—Mottling with air bronchogram
❏ Stage III—Heart border cannot delineated properly
❏ Stage IV—White out lung.

Differential Diagnosis of Hyaline Membrane Disease (Radiological)

❏ Meconium aspiration syndrome
❏ Total anomalous pulmonary venous connection
❏ Pulmonary hemorrhage
❏ Pulmonary edema
❏ Congenital pneumonia
❏ Stillbirth
❏ Laryngeal or tracheal atresia
❏ Congenital lymphangiectasia.

Case 29 (Fig. 8.38)

❏ A newborn with respiratory distress

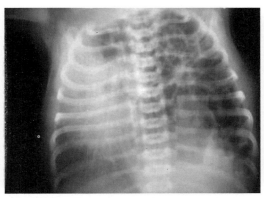

Fig. 8.38: Diaphragmatic hernia.

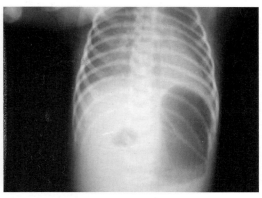

Fig. 8.40: Double bubble shadow: duodenal atresia.

❐ Radiograph showing diaphragmatic hernia (bowel loops in the chest, mediastinal shift to right, and absence of left dome of diaphragm).

Case 30 (Fig. 8.39)

❐ A newborn child brought dead.

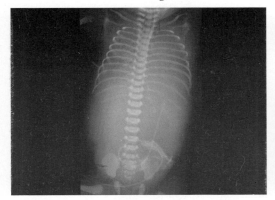

Fig. 8.39: Tracheo-esophageal atresia (no air in the lungs and stomach).

Case 31 (Fig. 8.40)

❐ Another newborn with respiratory distress, vomiting, and abdominal distension
❐ Radiograph showing double bubble shadow in the abdomen. It is a case of duodenal atresia.

Similar picture may be seen in a case of annular pancreas also. Note that lung fields are normal in this child with respiratory distress.

Case 32 (Fig. 8.41)

❐ A child with some abnormal findings on general examination

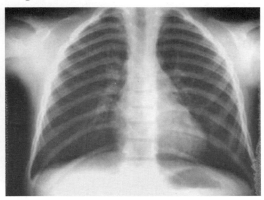

Fig. 8.41: Radiograph showing absence of clavicle.

❐ Radiograph showing absence of clavicle (a case of craniocleidodysostosis).

Case 33 (Fig. 8.42)

❐ Child with fever, cough, and breathlessness

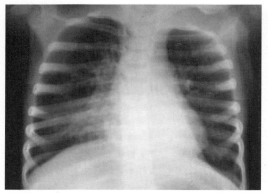

Fig. 8.42: Collapse of left lower lobe.

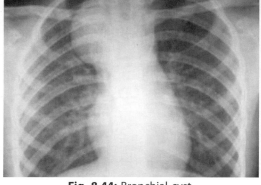

Fig. 8.44: Bronchial cyst.

❐ Collapse of left lower lobe.

Case 34 (Fig. 8.43)

❐ A child with sudden onset of dyspnea and chest pain

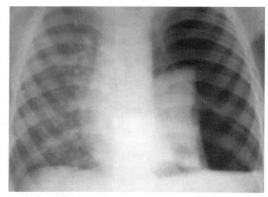

Fig. 8.43: Hydropneumothorax (left).

❐ X-ray showing hydropneumothorax on left.
Note the collapsed lung and mediastinal shift.

Case 35 (Figs. 8.44 and 8.45)

❐ A child with cough of long duration

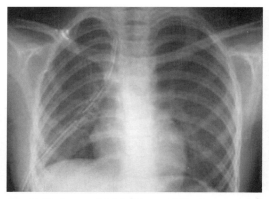

Fig. 8.45: Same child in Figure 8.32 after surgery.

❐ A case of bronchial cyst and it was surgically removed (drainage tube in situ).

Case 36 (Fig. 8.46)

❐ An 8-year-old girl with fever of 2 weeks duration
❐ Not very symptomatic. Treated with two courses of antibiotics. No response
❐ Cold agglutination test—positive
❐ Treated with erythromycin and improved
❐ It was a case of *Mycoplasma pneumoniae*
❐ Higher antibiotics may not be effective.

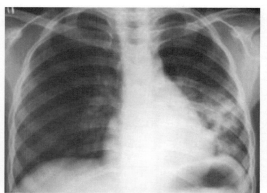

Fig. 8.46: Left lower pneumonia in an 8-year-old girl.

Case 37 (Fig. 8.47)

❏ A 12-year-old child with fever and cough

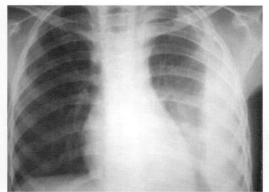

Fig. 8.47: Radiograph showing lamellar pleural effusion, responded to erythromycin.

❏ Radiograph showing pleural effusion, again due to *Mycoplasma pneumoniae*
❏ *Mycoplasma pneumoniae* may present with different radiological findings.

■ INTERESTING CARDIOLOGY CASES

Case 38 (Fig. 8.48)

❏ A 3-month-old child with cyanotic heart disease with dyspnea. Prominent jugular venous wave

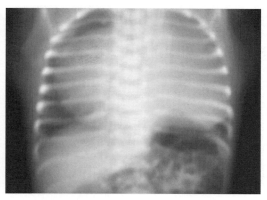

Fig. 8.48: Cardiomegaly with prominent right atrium: tricuspid atresia.

❏ X-ray: Cardiomegaly with prominent right atrium
❏ ECG showed large P wave
❏ Echo: Tricuspid atresia.

Case 39 (Fig. 8.49)

❏ Child with developmental delay and large head.

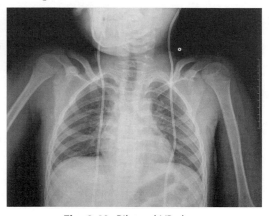

Fig. 8.49: Bilateral VP shunt

Case 40 (Fig. 8.50)

❏ A 3-year-old child with cyanosis. No features of heart failure
❏ Boot-shaped heart

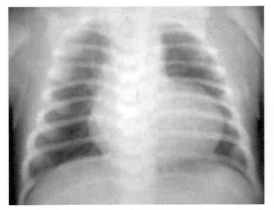

Fig. 8.50: Boot-shaped heart: Fallot's tetralogy.

- ❏ Fallot's tetralogy
- ❏ Other X-ray features of TOF include the following:
  - Absence of cardiomegaly
  - Pulmonary oligemia
  - Concave pulmonary bay
  - Right-sided aortic arch (in 25%).

Case 41 (Fig. 8.51)

- ❏ Child with recurrent cough and sinusitis

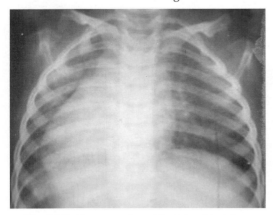

Fig. 8.51: Dextrocardia with right sided liver.

- ❏ Dextrocardia with right sided liver—situs inversus
- ❏ X-ray of paranasal sinuses showed sinusitis (Kartagener's syndrome).

Case 42 (Fig. 8.52)

- ❏ Otherwise asymptomatic child
- ❏ X-ray taken for right-sided apex beat

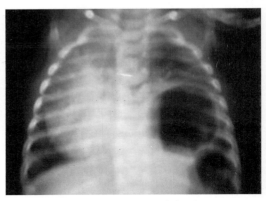

Fig. 8.52: Eventeration of diaphragm.

- ❏ Eventeration of diaphragm (dextraposition).

Case 43 (Fig. 8.53)

- ❏ Child with features of cardiac failure from early childhood
- ❏ On examination, grossly shifted apex beat

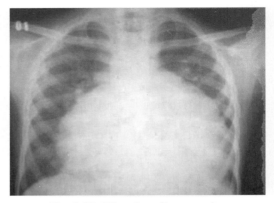

Fig. 8.53: Dilated cardiomyopathy.

- ❏ Echo: Dilated cardiomyopathy.

Case 44 (Fig. 8.54)

- ❐ A 9-year-old child from school health check-up
- ❐ On examination: Low volume femoral pulse, cardiomegaly, and short systolic murmur

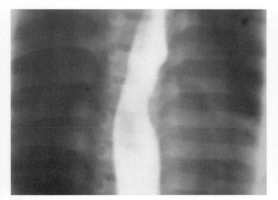

Fig. 8.54: Barium study showing inverted three appearance: coarctation of aorta.

- ❐ Barium study showed inverted three appearance
- ❐ X-ray chest of this child showed rib notching (three to nine ribs) also
- ❐ A case of coarctation of aorta.

Causes of Rib Notching

- ❐ Coarctation of aorta
- ❐ Neurofibroma
- ❐ Thalassemia major
- ❐ Collaterals in coronary heart disease
- ❐ Marfan syndrome
- ❐ AV fistula
- ❐ Blalock–Taussig surgery
- ❐ Idiopathic.

Case 45 (Figs. 8.55 and 8.56)

- ❐ A 4-month-old male child with history of severe breathlessness
- ❐ History of excessive crying during feeding and passing stool

- ❐ On examination: Dyspneic, low volume pulse cardiomegaly, S3, and Gr III systolic murmur
- ❐ Respiratory system: No air entry on left side
- ❐ Tender and soft hepatosplenomegaly

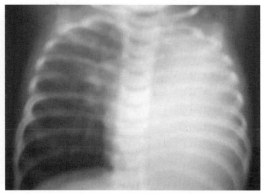

Fig. 8.55: Huge cardiomegaly: a case of anomalous left coronary artery arising from pulmonary artery (ALCAPA).

- ❐ X-ray showing huge cardiomegaly
- ❐ ECG showed ST segment elevation in L-1, aVL, and V_4-V_6 and Q wave in V_4-V_6
- ❐ Echo showed anomalous left coronary artery arising from pulmonary artery (ALCAPA), very poor left ventricular ejection fraction
- ❐ Child was treated with supporting measures and decongestive treatment

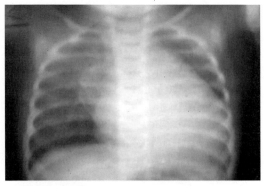

Fig. 8.56: Same child in Figure 8.55 after decongestive treatment.

❒ Gross reduction in cardiac size after decongestive treatment.

■ INTERESTING BONE X-RAYS

Case 46 (Figs. 8.57 and 8.58)

❒ A known case of cerebral palsy (CP) with fracture of right upper limb

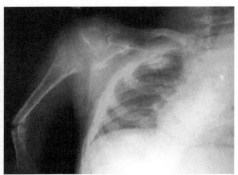

Fig. 8.57: Widening of humerus epiphysis: a case of rickets in a child with cerebral palsy.

❒ Widening of humerus epiphysis, poorly formed head, and osteoporosis. Promptly responded to vitamin D.

Rickets in CP may be due to:
❒ Dietary deficiency
❒ Anticonvulsant drug
❒ Poor exposure to sunlight
❒ Grossly restricted activity
❒ Radiograph of chest of another child with CP, again showing features of rickets on right humerus.

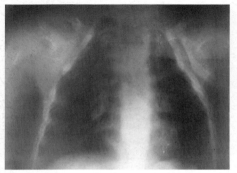

Fig. 8.58: Features of rickets with decreased bone density.

Case 47 (Fig. 8.59)

❒ A child with CHD underwent surgery.

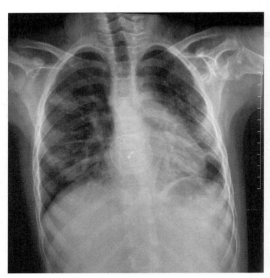

Fig. 8.59: ASD closure device (Amplatzer).

Case 48 (Fig. 8.60)

❒ Child with rickets, with pain on right forearm

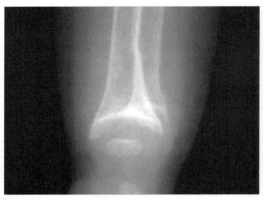

Fig. 8.60: Fracture of radius with features of rickets.

❒ Radiograph shows greenstick fracture of radius and features of rickets
❒ History of fall could not be elicited in this case.

Case 49 (Figs. 8.61 and 8.62)

❑ A 15-month-old child, not able to stand
❑ No history of birth asphyxia
❑ Sitting with support at 6 month, without support at 8 month, all other spheres of development—normal
❑ On examination: Active, doing all activities by sitting
❑ General and systemic examination—normal

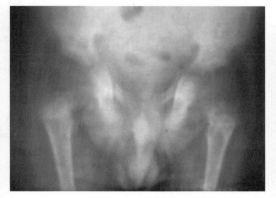

Fig. 8.61: X-ray pelvis with poorly formed head of the femur on both sides.

❑ Radiograph showing poorly formed head of the femur of both sides
❑ Diagnosed as case of rickets radiologically and biochemically
❑ Treated with vitamin D. After one-and-half-month child was able to walk

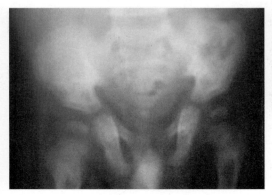

Fig. 8.62: Same child in Figure 8.54 after treatment with vitamin D.

❑ Repeat X-ray shows well-formed femoral head. This child did not have any other features of rickets.

Case 50 (Figs. 8.63 and 8.64)

❑ A 4-year-old girl, complaining of neck pain at the end of X-mas vacation
❑ Suspected school phobia
❑ All routine investigations were normal
❑ Treated with symptomatic measures, but no improvement

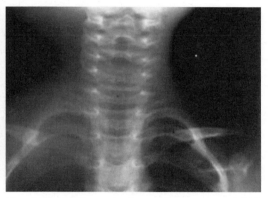

Fig. 8.63: Radiograph shows destruction of fifth cervical vertebra.

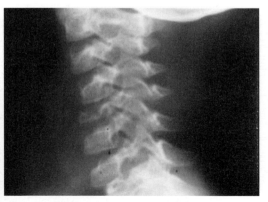

Fig. 8.64: Same child in Figure 8.56, lateral view: eosinophilic granuloma.

❑ Radiograph shows destruction of fifth cervical vertebra
❑ MRI and later biopsy proved it was case of eosinophilic granuloma.

Case 51 (Fig. 8.65)

❑ Known case of thalassemia on blood transfusion

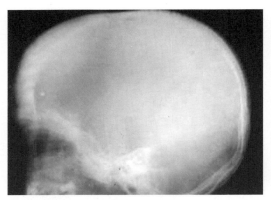

Fig. 8.65: Hair-on-end appearance: hemolytic anemia.

❑ Skull radiograph shows hair on end appearance.

Case 52 (Fig. 8.66)

❑ Swelling over right clavicle

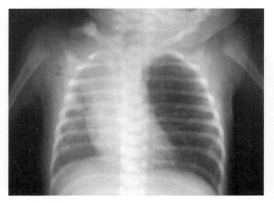

Fig. 8.66: Fracture of right clavicle.

❑ Fracture right clavicle. A history of fall could not be elicited in this case.

Case 53 (Fig. 8.67)

❑ Fever with skin rash
❑ History of knee joint pain after 1 month

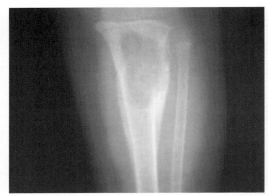

Fig. 8.67: Osteolytic lesion of the left tibia without surrounding sclerosis: histiocytosis.

❑ Radiograph shows osteolytic lesion of the left tibia without surrounding sclerosis
❑ Diagnosed as a case of histiocytosis.

Case 54 (Figs. 8.68 to 8.71)

❑ Radiographs of skull and long bones of different children showing osteolytic lesion suggestive of histiocytosis.

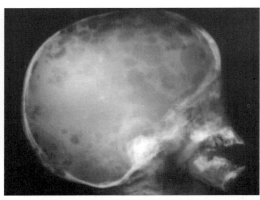

Fig. 8.68: Radiographs of skull showing osteolytic lesion suggestive of histiocytosis.

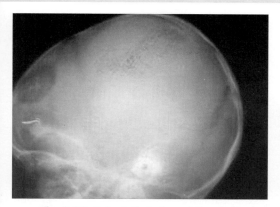

Fig. 8.69: Osteolytic lesion of the skull.

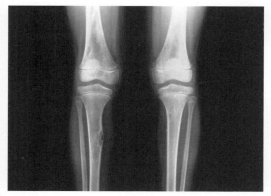

Fig. 8.70: Radiographs of femur and tibia showing osteolytic lesion suggestive of histiocytosis.

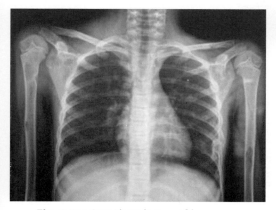

Fig. 8.71: Osteolytic lesion of humerus.

Case 55 (Figs. 8.72 and 8.73)

- ❏ Child referred as a case of "seizure"
- ❏ General examination showed shortening of fingers and toes

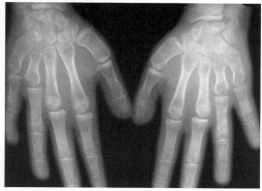

Fig. 8.72: Radiograph shows shortening of fourth and fifth metacarpals: a case of hypoparathyroidism.

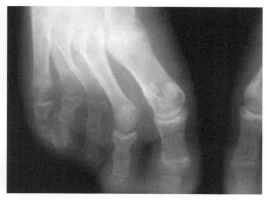

Fig. 8.73: Same child in Figure 8.65, showing shortening of fourth and fifth metatarsals.

- ❏ Radiograph shows shortening of fourth and fifth metacarpals and metatarsals.
- ❏ Investigations: Low calcium, high phosphorus, and low parathyroid hormone level
- ❏ It was a case of pseudohypoparathyroidism.

Case 56 (Figs. 8.74 to 8.76)

❏ Child with severe anemia and hepatosplenomegaly

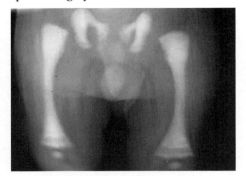

Fig. 8.74: Osteopetrorickets.

❏ It is a case of osteopetrosis. In this case,
there are features of rickets also (Osteopetrorickets)

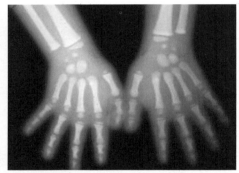

Fig. 8.75: Radiograph shows increased bone
density: osteopetrosis.

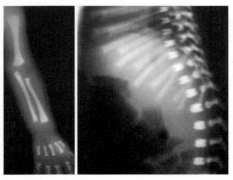

Fig. 8.76: Generalized increase in bone density:
osteopetrosis.

❏ Radiograph shows increased bone density
❏ No corticomedullary differentiation is seen.

Case 57 (Fig. 8.77)

❏ Child with headache and vomiting

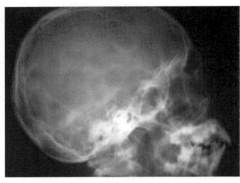

Fig. 8.77: Skull radiograph showing silver beaten
appearance.

❏ Skull radiograph shows silver beaten appearance, suggestive of raised intracranial
tension (ICT)
❏ Other features of raised ICT include
separation of sutures, erosion of posterior
clinoid process, and scalloping of pituitary
fossa.

Case 58 (Fig. 8.78)

❏ A 12-year-old boy with juvenile chronic
rheumatoid arthritis with marked deformity

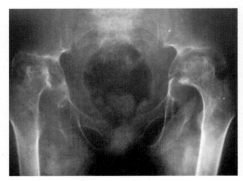

Fig. 8.78: Bilateral destruction of both femoral head
and roof of the acetabulum: a case of juvenile rheumatoid arthritis (JRA).

❏ Radiograph shows bilateral destruction of both femoral head and roof of the acetabulum (bony ankylosis).

Case 59 (Figs. 8.79 and 8.80)

❏ A 4-year male child with recurrent lower abdominal pain. General practitioner ordered X-ray pelvis

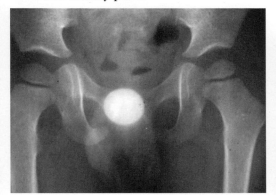

Fig. 8.79: Radiograph shows dense rounded shadow: penile shadow in anteroposterior direction.

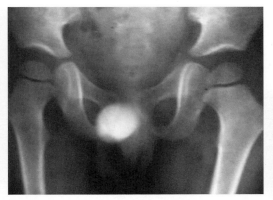

Fig. 8.80: Same child in Figure 8.72, with change in position.

❏ Radiograph shows dense rounded shadow. Shadow almost same in repeated X-rays
❏ No history of foreign body ingestion
❏ Otherwise, child was asymptomatic and all other investigations were normal

❏ Radiograph repeated in a different position
❏ Repeated radiograph failed to show the same shadow. The dense rounded opacity is due to penile shadow.

Case 60 (Figs. 8.81 and 8.82)

❏ A 4-year-old boy with weakness of both lower limbs since birth and incontinence of urine and stool. No history of trauma or injection

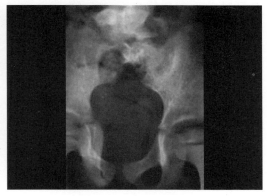

Fig. 8.81: Sacral agenesis.

❏ Radiograph shows sacral agenesis
❏ Late intravenous pyelogram (IVP) showed left renal agenesis (IVP advised based on ultrasonogram abdomen).

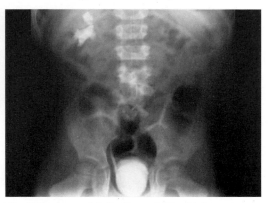

Fig. 8.82: Same child in Figure 8.74 with intravenous pyelogram showing left renal agenesis.

❏ Final diagnosis: Sacral agenesis with agenesis of left kidney.

Case 61 (Fig. 8.83)

❏ A child with transfusion-dependent anemia and history of minor fall.

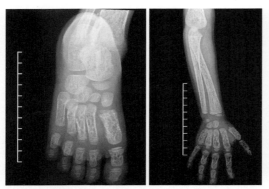

Fig. 8.83: A case of thalassemia and severe osteoporosis.

Case 62 (Fig. 8.84)

❏ A child with difficulty in holding clothes or wooden bar.

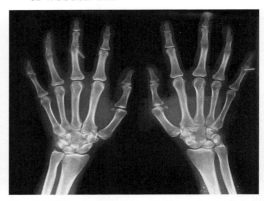

Fig. 8.84: Symphalangism of bilateral middle and ring finger.

Bibliography

1. Amplatz K, Moller JH. Radiology of Congenital Heart Disease. Mosby Year Book; 2001.
2. Bettmann MA. The chest radiograph in cardiovascular disease. In: Bonow RO, Mann DL, Zipes DP, Libby P (Eds). Braunwald's Heart Disease, 9th edition. Elsevier; 2012.
3. Cooley RN, Schriber MH. Radiology of the Heart & Great Vessels, 3rd edition. Williams & Wilkins; 1979.
4. Carty H, Brunelle F, Shaw D, Kendall B. Imaging Children. New York: Churchill Livingstone; 1994.
5. De Hauwere A, Bacher K, Smeets P, et al. Analysis of image quality in digital chest imaging. Radiat Prot Dosimetry. 2005;117(1–3):174-77.
6. Dobbins JT, Godfrey DJ, McAdams HP. Chest tomosynthesis. Syllabus RSNA 2003, Advances in digital radiography: RSNA categorical course in diagnostic radiology physics. 2003; 211-17.
7. Fryback DG, Thornbury JR. The efficacy of diagnostic imaging. Medical Descision Making. 1991;11(2):88-94.
8. Greulich WW, Pyle SI. Radiographic Atlas of Skeletal Development of Hand and Wrist. Stanford: Stanford University Press; 1950 (reprint 1954).
9. Hullet RL, Ovitt TW. The chest roentgenogram. In: Allen HD, Gutagesell HP, Clark EB, Driscoll DJ (Eds). Moss & Adams Heart Disease in Infants, Children and Adolescents, 6th edition. Lippincott Williams & Wilkins; 2001.
10. Jefferson K, Rees S. Clinical Cardiac Radiology, 2nd edition. London & Boston: Butterworths; 1980.
11. Kozlowski K, Beighton P. Gamut Index of Skeletal Dysplasias: An Aid to Radiodiagnosis. Berlin: Springer-Verlag; 1984. pp. 182-9.
12. Kuhn, Slovis, Haller. Caffey's Pediatric Diagnostic Imaging, 10th edition. New York: Mosby; 2004.
13. Robert O'Rourke, Walsh R, Fuster V. Cardiac roentgenography. Hurst's The Manual of Cardiology. 12th edition. Mc Graw Hill; 2008.
14. Singleton EB, Morriss MJH. Plan radiographic diagnosis of CHD. In: Gorson A, Bricker JT, Fisher DJ, New SR (Eds). The Science & Practice of Pediatric Cardiology, 2nd edition. Williams & Wilkins; 1998.
15. Swischuk LE. Plain Film Interpretation in Congenital Heart Diseases. Lea & Febiger; 1970.
16. Swischuk LE. Differential Diagnosis in Pediatric Radiology. Philadelphia: Lippincott Williams & Wilkins; 1995.
17. Tanner JM, Whitehouse RH, Marshall WA, et al. Assessment of skeletal maturity and prediction of adult height. London: Academic Press,; 1975.
18. Taybi H, Lachman RS. Radiology of syndromes, metabolic disorders, and skeletal dysplasias, 4th edition. Chicago: Mosby-Year Book; 1996.

Index

Page numbers followed by *f* refer to figure and *t* refer to table.